ALSO BY BOB GREENE

The Best Life Diet Daily Journal

Bob Greene's Total Body Makeover

Bob Greene's Total Body Makeover Daily Journal

The Get with the Program! Guide to Fast Food & Family Restaurants

The Get with the Program! Guide to Good Eating

The Get with the Program! Daily Journal

Get with the Program!

Make the Connection: Ten Steps to a Better Body—and a Better Life

A Journal of Daily Renewal: The Companion to Make the Connection

Keep the Connection: Choices for a Better Body and a Better Life

BOB GREENE
THE BEST

LIFE DIET

SIMON & SCHUSTER PAPERBACKS
NEW YORK   LONDON   TORONTO   SYDNEY

This publication contains the opinions and ideas of its author. It is intended to provide helpful and informative material on the subjects addressed in the publication. It is sold with the understanding that the author and publisher are not engaged in rendering medical, health, psychological, or any other kind of personal professional services in the book. If the reader requires personal medical, health, or other assistance or advice, a competent professional should be consulted.

The author and publisher specifically disclaim all responsibility for any liability, loss, or risk, personal or otherwise, that is incurred as a consequence, directly or indirectly, of the use and application of any of the contents of this book.

Before starting on a weight-loss plan, or beginning or modifying an exercise program, check with your physician to make sure that the changes are right for you

SIMON & SCHUSTER PAPERBACKS
1230 Avenue of the Americas
New York, NY 10020

Copyright © 2006 by the Bestlife Corporation
Photographs copyright © 2006 by Alan Richardson

Photographer: Alan Richardson. Food Stylist: Michael Pederson.
Prop Stylist: Debrah E. Donahue

First Simon & Schuster trade paperback edition December 2007

SIMON & SCHUSTER PAPERBACKS and colophon are registered trademarks of Simon & Schuster, Inc.

For information about special discounts for bulk purchases, please contact Simon & Schuster Special Sales at 1-800-456-6798 or business@simonandschuster.com

Designed by Joel Avirom and Jason Snyder

Manufactured in the United States of America

10 9 8 7 6 5 4 3 2 1

Library of Congress Control Number: 2006052222

ISBN-13: 978-1-4165-4066-3
ISBN-10:   1-4165-4066-0
ISBN-13: 978-1-4165-4069-4 (pbk)
ISBN-10:   1-4165-4069-5 (pbk)

The author gratefully acknowledges permission from the following source to reprint material in their control: "Morning Prayer," from Illuminata by Marianne Williamson, copyright © 1994 by Marianne Williamson. Used by permission of Random House, Inc.

ACKNOWLEDGMENTS

▶ Special thanks to Daryn Eller; Janis Jibrin, M.S., R.D.; Susan B. Dopart, M.S., R.D.; Karen Gillingham, Sara Kate Gillingham-Ryan, Carolyn O'Neil, M.S., R.D.; Liz Weiss, M.S., R.D.; Janice Newell Bissex, M.S., R.D.; John J. Merendino Jr., M.D.; Amy L. Anderson; Tracy Olgeaty Gensler, M.S., R.D.; Sidra Forman; and Heather K. Jones, R.D.

CONTENTS

FOREWORD

▶ I feel like I've always known Bob Greene, though the truth is, it's only been fourteen years since we first met. My life has not been the same since that meeting; Bob changed my life.

At the time, I was 237 pounds, miserable and so ashamed to have joined the ranks of the perpetually obese that I had trouble maintaining eye contact. I couldn't understand why I was able to triumph over so many other challenges and adversities in life, and yet when it came to losing weight I was a big fat failure.

Before I met Bob, I had spent years bouncing from one diet to another, beginning from the time I was twenty-two. That was the year that I landed a big job as a news coanchor in Baltimore and discovered that food—and especially corn dogs and six-inch chocolate-chip cookies with macadamia nuts from the mall food stalls—could provide a great deal of solace. I was naïve, felt very alone, and was having trouble adjusting to my new job.

I had no friends and no furniture, not even curtains on the windows of my new apartment. My coanchor seemed to resent me, and I worried that I was in way over my head. I'd had almost no experience as a writer, but every day I was given news copy to rewrite for my segment of the broadcast. In my previous job I had been more of a newsreader: the copy had been written for me and all I had to do was read it on air. It's an awful feeling when you know you can't make the mark. No matter how hard I tried, I could not bang out the copy fast enough for my superiors. Inevitably, every day as we neared the six o'clock news hour I'd hear John, the copy editor, yell across the room: "WINFREY, WHERE'S THE GODDAMNED COPY!!!!"

I was humiliated but put on a smile and got through the days, reading the news and chitchatting with my fellow anchors on air. But I didn't like my job. I felt blessed to have it, but I truly hated some of the things I was required to do. I always felt like I was chasing bodies, waiting for the worst to happen. The bigger the fire, the more bodies in the collision, the more devastating the natural disaster, the more excited my bosses became.

Working in that environment was an affront to my spirit; the reporter's objectivity I needed to maintain went against everything in my nature. Many times I was an eyewitness to the most devastating moments in people's lives, but I was not allowed to express any emotion. So I ate those emotions, and along with them, just about everything I could buy at the food court. I thought I was just fine; I just had a little weight problem. Now I realize I didn't have a weight problem. I had problems that I was burying by eating, but it wasn't until years later, after many conversations with Bob, that I finally made the connection.

When all those corn dogs and chocolate-chip cookies finally pushed me up to 140 pounds—a weight I would do the hula in the streets for now—I went to my first diet doctor. I paid $27 for a consultation and an eating plan that called for 1,200 calories a day. It was my first time counting and cutting calories, so of course my young body responded well. I lost 7 pounds the first week, and in a month I was down to 125. Slim again, I started my old habit of grazing through the food stalls at the mall. My regular dinner plan: a baked potato with all the toppings—melted cheese, bacon, and chives—followed by one of those six-inch cookies from the Great American Cookies stand. In my freezer were stacks of Stouffer's macaroni and cheese, my comfort food of choice.

And so it went. I'd gain some, then I'd lose some. It was a cycle I'd end up repeating again and again.

When I first met Bob and he asked me why I was overweight, I thought he was being a smart-ass. I was overweight for the same reason everybody else is, I answered smugly. I loved food.

It took me a while to get to the truth. I didn't love food. I used food to numb my negative feelings. It didn't matter what the feeling was. A phone call from someone I didn't want to talk to; a confrontation of any kind; being late; feeling tired, anxious, or bored. No matter how insignificant the discomfort, my first reaction was to reach for something to eat: a grape, Cheerios, a handful of nuts, chips, popcorn. I'd eat, unaware of how much I was consuming, until I was chewing on the last kernels of corn. That's what it means to live unconsciously.

What I know for sure is that living an unconscious life is like being the walking dead. All my fat years—my unconscious years—are a blur to me now. It's only because I have photographs and diaries that I remember them at all. And sometimes even then I don't remember being present, because I wasn't really there.

I grew up believing that people with money didn't have problems. Or certainly none that money couldn't solve. Then, in 1986, my show went national. It changed the trajectory of my life. When I'd started my working life in Nashville and Baltimore, paying the rent and the electric bill and making payments on my car left me with just enough to buy groceries and get my hair done. Now I had more money than I'd ever imagined, and everybody wanted some. The first thing I did was to retire my mother and a cousin who helped take care of me when I was growing up. My father let me buy him a new house and a Mercedes, but he refused to quit working in his barbershop. He's still there.

Then everybody came out of the woodwork. Distant family members, who I barely knew, wanted me to completely take care of them or wanted to work for me. Relatives I hadn't seen since I was ten years old showed up demanding thousands of dollars "because we're family." Helping my family was something I wanted to do, but I didn't know how to handle the total strangers who came to Chicago claiming to have spent their last dime leaving a battering spouse, or the teenagers who'd run away from home.

The first year I helped almost everyone who asked me, family and strangers alike. It was stressful trying to figure out how much to give to whom, and before I knew it, they'd return for more. I was overwhelmed, but I never felt it. Once again, I just ate until I couldn't feel. By the end of the year I was 200 pounds.

In 1988, totally frustrated and up to 212 pounds, I turned to Optifast, a liquid diet supplement program. For four months, I ate not a single grape, nut, or other morsel of food. I lost fat—and muscle—and I dropped to 145 pounds.

Now I know that it's impossible to starve your body for four months, then feed it, and not expect to regain the weight. Your body doesn't want to starve, so it holds on to every ounce of fat in case you do another crazy thing like consuming only about 400 calories a day!

It would take seven more years of gaining, gaining, and countless attempts to follow diets that I wasn't really prepared to stick to before I discovered the truth. In the meantime, I was racing through two hundred shows a year. My entire life was work. I was leaving my apartment at six A.M. and getting home at ten at night. Eating. Sleeping. Repeating the cycle five days a week. My friends were my staff, and even when we weren't working, our lives still revolved around the show.

In 1992, I won another Emmy for Best Talk Show Host. I had prayed that Phil Donahue would win so that I wouldn't have to embarrass myself by rolling my fat butt out of my seat and walking down the aisle to the stage. By now I'd reached the end of believing I could be thin, though I was scheduled to leave for Colorado the next day to visit yet another spa. I was so depressed about my weight, I had little hope that I would be successful this time around. Every time the number on the scale went higher, it seemed even more hopeless. And 237 pounds was the heaviest I'd ever been. I had journals filled with prayers to God to help me conquer my weight demon.

Bob Greene was the answer to my prayers. When I first met Bob at that last-ditch-effort spa in Colorado, I thought for sure he was judging and labeling me as I had already judged and labeled myself: fat and out of control. Bob, it turned out, wasn't judging me at all. He really understood.

But he did have some tough questions for me. One of them was the hardest question that anyone has ever asked me: What is the best life possible for you? I remember one conversation in particular.

"You of all the people in the world can have your life be what you want; why don't you do it? What do you really want?" he asked.

"I want to be happy," I replied.

"'Happy' isn't a good-enough answer. What does that mean? Break it down for me. When was the last time you were really happy?"

"When I was filming *The Color Purple*, seven years ago."

"What about filming *The Color Purple* made you happy?"

I didn't have to think to answer. "Doing that work filled me up. I was playing a character that was meaningful to me, surrounded by the brilliance of Alice Walker, Quincy Jones, and Steven Spielberg. I was so charged and stimulated every day, I just wanted to do better and be better."

"So what would it take for you to have that feeling again?"

In answering that question, I realized the show had gotten away from me. In order to stay competitive, we had become more and more salacious, covering topics like "My sister slept with my husband" and "Is my husband or my boss my baby's father?" I didn't want to put junk on the air that perpetuated dysfunction instead of resolving it. It wasn't who I wanted to be.

And so, while I worked out and changed what and how much I ate, managing the rest of my life became my real focus. I started asking myself the same questions Bob had asked me. For every circumstance, I asked myself:

"What do I want?"

"What kind of show do I want?"

"What kind of body do I want?"

"What do I want to give to all the people who are asking me for my money, my attention, my time?"

I finally made a decision about that last one. I set up trust funds with a finite amount of cash for the people to whom I wanted to give money. And to those with whom I had no connection, I said no, and meant it. And just to be sure, I changed my home number. I've never visited a psychiatrist, but working with Bob has been priceless therapy.

Another thing I know for sure now is that you've got to ask yourself: What kind of life do *I* want and how close am I to living it? You cannot ever live the life of your dreams without coming face to face with the truth. Every unwanted pound creates another layer of lies. It's only when you peel back those layers that you will be set free: free to work out, free to eat responsibly, free to live the life you want and deserve to live. Tell the truth and you'll learn to eat to satisfy your physical hunger as opposed to your emotional hunger and to stop burying your hopes and dreams beneath layers of fat.

A young woman on my show who had been struggling with her weight once said to me she'd learned to challenge the pain and not the peanut butter. I thought that was brilliant. Once you work on what's eating you, you won't want to eat so much.

The Best Life Diet plan on the following pages mirrors the way I eat and live now. (You'll find a full week of my menus and some of my favorite foods on pages 161–167.) There is no secret to losing weight. It's simple physics: what you put in versus what you put out.

I lost weight in stages. First I became active: I still work out even though I really hate it, but I know if I don't, I will end up at 200 pounds again. Then I started working on my eating. First I stopped eating past 7:30 at night. When Bob told me it would make a big difference in my weight, I resisted. I thought it was going to be too hard. It was at first, but it gradually got easier. I rearranged my life so I wasn't rushing to make the 7:30 P.M. eating cutoff time. Not eating after 7:30 P.M. turned out to be one of the most effective changes I've made.

I've now taken most of the unhealthy foods out of my diet and replaced them with better choices. I eat smaller portions and healthful foods as a way of life, not as a diet to go on and off. I've even started a garden, and one of the most delightful moments for me these days is seeing a basket of just-picked green beans, tomatoes, lettuce, carrots, and corn sitting on my kitchen counter. And I'm always working on getting better. My diet is a work in progress.

Maybe what's most different now is that I think about *why* I eat, not just about what and how much. The truth is, most people—like me— have to keep watch on all three: why, what, and how we eat. We have to manage it daily. If you turn on the TV and see that I've picked up a few pounds, you will know that I'm not managing and balancing my life as well as I should.

I accept that mine is a very public life, although the pain and frustration I experience when I gain weight is just as individual and difficult as your own. I still work constantly at not repressing my feelings with food.

One day I was leaving Santa Barbara, heading for Chicago. I was unable to fly due to bad weather, and I left the airport craving cake. I didn't process my feelings about being delayed; I just wanted cake. In particular, the coconut cake sold at the Montecito Café. Mind you, it was three years ago that I had my first and last bite of that cake, but the memory was so strong I could taste it. All the way home I thought about that cake.

I knew the café was closed, but I was still obsessing about it. I got home and stood in my pantry trying to come up with something that would substitute for the cake and satisfy my craving. I got out some pancake mix and a can of pineapple. I can make pineapple pancakes, add syrup, and it can taste kind of like the cake, I thought. I vowed to make a giant pancake right after I took my dogs for a walk.

While the dogs and I went for a long walk, I got really calm. I wasn't anxious about missing appointments and having to rearrange schedules anymore. I returned home and didn't even think about cake or pancakes, pineapple or syrup.

I started a new book, and went to sleep in peace.

Pausing is something I do more often now.

And I pray or meditate—or do both—every day. I start my day with a prayer that Marianne Williamson shared in her book *Illuminata: A Return to Prayer.*

> *Dear God,*
> *I give this day to You.*
> *May my mind stay centered on the things of spirit.*
> *May I not be tempted to stray from love.*
> *As I begin this day, I open to receive You.*
> *Please enter where You already abide.*
> *May my mind and heart be pure and true, and may I not deviate*
>   *from the things of goodness.*
> *May I see the love and innocence in all mankind, behind the masks*
>   *we all wear and the illusions of this worldly plane.*
> *I surrender to You my doings this day.*
> *I ask only that they serve You and the healing of the world.*
> *May I bring Your love and goodness with me, to give unto others*
>   *wherever I go.*
> *Make me the person You would have me be.*
> *Direct my footsteps, and show me what You would have me do.*
> *Make the world a safer, more beautiful place.*
> *Bless all Your creatures.*
> *Heal us all, and use me, dear Lord, that I might know the joy of being*
>   *used by You.*
> *Amen.*

I pray to be used by a power greater than myself. It takes consistent effort to live my best life.

The mistake I've made in the past is not realizing how constant a struggle it really is not to turn to food for comfort. It comes down to another question Bob asked me years ago: "How much do you love yourself?"

"Of course I love myself," I'd snapped. "It's the first law of self-preservation. I firmly believe in it."

"You may believe it, but you don't practice it," he said. "Otherwise you couldn't let yourself be two hundred and thirty-seven pounds."

I wanted to cry, and later I did. He was so right. I cared more about everyone else's feelings than my own. I'd overextend myself to do anything anyone asked, to honor his or her feelings. I didn't want anyone to think I wasn't "nice" or, worse, that "the money has gone to her head."

This, too, I know for sure: Loving yourself means honoring yourself and your own feelings *first*. When I was 237 pounds, I didn't even know what I felt. It was like living behind a veil of fat.

My hope is that you can learn from my mistakes and liberate yourself from this struggle. I finally know it doesn't have to be so hard. Make a decision. Know that you deserve the best life possible. It's there for the asking, the answering, the taking. Go out and get it!!!!!

INTRODUCTION

▶ Losing weight is not that complicated. Eat fewer calories than you burn and the pounds will drop off, your clothes will loosen up, and you'll see a lower number on the scale. It's that simple. Only it never really is that simple. While the formula for weight loss may be uncomplicated, people are not. To varying degrees, we're all at the mercy of our physical yearnings, years of deeply ingrained habits, roller-coaster emotions, social pressures, and an inborn penchant for pleasure—in short, we all have our own human nature to contend with, and that has turned the relatively straight-forward process of losing weight into a surprisingly complex problem.

When you're faced with complex problems in other areas of your life, you probably think nothing of devoting much of your time to resolving them. After all, common wisdom has it that if you approach a challenge by taking it step by step, success will come. However, weight loss is rarely ap-proached that way. Most people want immediate gratification, and so most weight-loss programs try to deliver. They ask you to jump in and ruthlessly cut your calories so that you drop pounds right away. A few weeks later, they let you ease up and eat more, then a few weeks after that you can ease up again, until it's easier and easier to relax the rules and you find yourself eating and living the same way you did before you went on the diet. As a result, you gain back all the weight you lost.

The quick-fix approach has always seemed backward to me. If there's any doubt that making drastic changes to behavior in the short term is no way to approach a multifaceted problem, you only have to look at the diet failure rates in this country. Despite spending billions of dollars on weight-loss plans and paraphernalia, not all that many people are getting to a healthy weight permanently. But *some* people are, and most of them are doing it not by asking the impossible of themselves—and, for most people, rapid transformation that *lasts* is impossible—but by taking change one small step at a time. These people increase the amount of physical activity they're doing and stop skipping meals. They look at their lives and work on changing the reasons why they turn to food for comfort. They learn how to get in better touch with their hunger, and, finally, they embrace a new, more moderate and nutritious way of eating. Doing *all* of these things, and doing them in a gradual way, is what enables these people to reach and maintain healthy body weights. It's the reverse of the quick-fix approach—and it really works!

I'm an exercise physiologist, so I've had a lot of training in how the human body operates. But my real education has come from being a student of diet successes and failures. Ever since I finished graduate school in 1983, I've been fascinated by how some people are able to lose weight and keep it off and how some people can't seem to make weight loss stick. This fascination has led me to make finding the answer to that question my life's work. *How* you lose weight is no great mystery—that's just a matter of eating fewer calories than you burn. The more puzzling question is *why*, after managing to shed at least some—or perhaps even a lot of—weight, so many people change course and return to their old ways. Even more puzzling is that when I ask people who've been on the weight-loss roller coaster how they felt when they were thinner, most of them say, "Great. I never felt better in my life." So what makes them regress?

After working one-on-one with many clients and talking to thousands of people through the years, I think I can say with some authority that the fast-and-furious approach to weight loss is also the fastest route to failure.

Here's why: human beings don't respond well to sudden changes. However, your body—and your mind—both have a powerful ability to adapt to change when it comes at you in measured amounts. Think about how athletes train. They don't immediately go from lifting 20 pounds to lifting 100 pounds, and they don't go from running 2 miles to running 26 miles overnight. Instead, they work up to the pinnacle of their capabilities, giving their bodies a chance to become accustomed to the new demands being placed on them. This step-by-step strategy makes sense when it comes to weight loss, too.

Change—or, I should say, lasting change—just takes time. And that's not only true of how our bodies work, it's also true of how our minds work. If you've always relied on food for emotional sustenance, you will have to get used to the idea of turning to other things to help you through tough times. Perhaps most important, you've got to figure out *why* you need food to make yourself feel better. What in your life is making you unhappy, or leaving a void that you're using ice cream and doughnuts to fill? If you're eating because you're stressed, angry, bored, or lonely, you've got to find out what's at the root of those feelings and change it. That may take some time, but it's one of the most critical components of weight loss. For Oprah, becoming aware of and dealing with her habit of burying her emotions under plates of food was *the* most critical component. For many people, it will be as well.

A BETTER WAY OF EATING, A BETTER WAY OF LIFE

The Best Life Diet is not a diet in the usual sense of the word. You don't go on it, then off it, as the term *diet* typically implies. It is, instead, a diet in the traditional sense of the word: a way of eating—for life. It's based on a well-balanced regimen of interesting, satisfying, nutrient-rich, and easy-to-find-and-prepare foods. It's not extremely restrictive in calories or limited in variety, but rather it is rooted in the idea that eating is and always should be one of life's greatest pleasures. You can love food and live happily on this diet while still meeting your weight-loss goals.

The bounty of wonderful food available to us is a blessing, and a curse. When you think about the sheer number of vegetables, fruits, grains, meats, oils, dairy products, nuts, legumes, and seeds available to us, it's mind-boggling. Run all those selections through the kitchens of food manufacturers and restaurants, and the choices expand thousands of times over. When you're trying to eat as healthfully as possible, that can make your head spin.

I want to make eating well as uncomplicated for you as possible while helping you to enjoy the great variety of foods out there. It's essential that you set certain boundaries for what you do and don't eat. This doesn't mean you have to deprive yourself; it just means that you have to opt for quality and wholesomeness. Choose whole grain cereal that is low in sugar instead of cereal that contains barely a hint of fiber and is sweetened to the hilt. Go for a lean turkey burger instead of a burger made from fat-marbled ground beef, and sparkling water spiked with real fruit juice instead of a fruit drink loaded with sugar.

This may be a new way of thinking for you, and I am keenly aware that when you're used to the intense flavor of one food, substitutes seem to pale in comparison. But I am just as aware of the fact that when you choose high-quality substitutes, your taste will change within a matter of weeks. This is key because what I'm asking you to do here is not to switch over to foods that are flavorless or bland, but foods that are really wonderful—they just happen to be good for you, too. There's nothing boring about a turkey burger spread with spicy mustard, smothered in onions that have been caramelized in a touch of olive oil, and served on a chewy whole grain bun. There's nothing dull about bubbly water splashed with tangy-sweet grapefruit juice and mango nectar or about many of the crunchy, nutty high-fiber O's and squares now being produced by cereal makers. These are the foods that are going to help you change your eating habits forever—and they're out there. You can buy them, and you can make them. Either way, they're going to make a big difference in your life.

I'm going to be honest—there *are* things you are going to have to give up. This program is going to help you eliminate foods that have empty calories as well as many that are filled with unhealthy fats, sugar, and artificial ingredients. But one glance at the recipes starting on page 191 should tell you that the enticing foods I'm going to ask you to replace them with will make it considerably easier to let the junky foods go.

Ideally, all of us would have access to beautiful, fresh vegetables and fruits all year round, and the time to prepare cooked-from-scratch meals every day. But most of us don't live where ripe peaches are available (or affordable) in January, and our busy lives mean that sometimes we're eating on the go. That's why being able to easily find foods that are convenient *and* healthy is crucial.

One way I hope to make it easier for you is by placing the Best Life Diet seal of approval that you see on the cover of this book on products that I believe meet the needs of anyone trying to lose weight and eat healthfully. The companies that offer these products have shown a commitment to removing or substantially reducing ingredients that aren't in your best interest, including saturated fats, trans fats, sodium, and sugar. Their products all contain one or more of the following nutritious ingredients: whole grains, healthy fats, fiber, vitamins, minerals, phytonutrients, and other essential nutrients. They're proof that it's not necessary to sacrifice great taste and nutrition to convenience, and they're readily available at supermarkets across the country.

The Best Life Diet seal helps you spot nutritious mainstays for meals and snacks. But what would life be like without a little ice cream, a piece of chocolate, or other treats? I firmly believe that you *should* eat these foods to make your diet fun and prevent feelings of deprivation. I've learned through the years that people who don't treat themselves aren't successful at losing and maintaining weight. The key, of course, is moderation. That's why I've put the Best Life Approved Treat seal on products that are individually portioned, have no more than 150 calories per serving, and tend to have a health edge over other treats in their class.

Florida Grapefruit and the Mushroom Council are two organizations that represent products bearing a Best Life seal of approval. You'll also find a seal on a wide variety of brands from General Mills, Unilever, and other companies. Look for a Best Life seal on Yoplait yogurt; Progresso soups; an array of products from Green Giant, Cascadian Farm organic, and Muir Glen organic; Bertolli olive oil; Lipton tea; Flatout wraps; 8th Continent soymilk; Barilla PLUS and Barilla whole grain pastas; Cheerios, Fiber One, Wheaties, and Total cereals; Wasa crispbread; Wish-Bone Salad Spritzers; Hellmann's (Best Food's) light and canola mayonnaise; One-A-Day Women's, Men's Health Formula, and 50 Plus multivitamins; Slim-Fast bars and shakes; Lean Cuisine; Skinny Cow; Edy's and Dreyer's Fruit Bars; and Libby's 100% Pure Pumpkin. I'm grateful to these companies and organizations for showing product innovation and concern for good health, and for supporting the Best Life Diet program.

THE BEST LIFE DIET BASICS

A primary goal of the Best Life Diet is to help you lose weight. But the program also has a more far-reaching purpose: to make sure that the pounds you lose don't return and your diet remains full of healthful, wholesome foods and virtually free of empty calories long past the time you reach your weight-loss goals. In other words, you're going to transform your diet not only long enough to slim down, but also for the rest of your life.

I believe, however, that dietary changes last only if you support those changes by first making some important investments in yourself. The Best Life Diet involves working on other things besides the foods that you eat, and each of those things—which include increasing your activity, understanding and gauging your hunger, and eliminating emotional eating—is going to shore up your efforts to cut calories and improve the quality of your diet. In my experience, all the modifications required by this plan play an indispensable role in long-term weight loss. They allow you to lay a solid foundation for dietary change, making it easier for you to alter your eating habits and increasing the likelihood of your success.

To follow this program, it's not necessary to count calories, follow menu plans, or measure your food. You can if you like—all the information you need to do so is provided on pages 125 and 126 and in the back of the book—and I know that those of you who prefer a structured plan or who have conditions that make weight loss particularly difficult can benefit from looking at and following the numbers. But you are also going to be adopting some practices that will help you gauge how much you should eat without consulting a chart. Learning to monitor your hunger, in particular, is going to provide you with cues that will let you know when you need to stop eating. Ultimately, I want eating the right amount of food for both weight loss and weight maintenance to come naturally to you so that you don't have to live your life tied to measuring cups and calorie counting.

The Best Life Diet is divided into three phases; the first two phases last at least four weeks, while the final one is open-ended. One reason that I'm not throwing everything at you at once is so that you don't become overwhelmed—as I said earlier, taking things step-by-step generally yields better results in any kind of endeavor, and particularly when it comes to weight loss. But there's also another reason that I'm going to ask you to make changes in stages. There's a logical order to the way your body adapts to new habits, and the three tiers of this program are designed to capitalize on that. The sequence in which you adopt changes during this program is not random; rather, it's intended to help you turn your body into a better weight-loss machine.

During Phase One, you're going to focus primarily on moving your body more and changing your eating patterns. You're barely going to alter what you eat during the initial weeks, so this is probably unlike diet programs you've tried before. There's a good reason why I'm going to have you hold off on overhauling the foods you eat: increasing your activity and restructuring your meals and snacks will rev up your metabolism, which will counter some of the problems you may otherwise bump up against when you begin cutting calories in earnest (cutting calories happens in Phase Two). The changes you make in Phase One will also help you regulate your appetite more effectively, and that will enhance your ability to handle the challenges to come.

During Phase Two, you will aggressively go after losing those extra pounds. You'll begin by making a few simple modifications to your diet, eliminating six foods that can inhibit weight loss. You will also learn about both the physical and emotional reasons why you get hungry, and you will begin employing tactics, including the use of a valuable tool called the hunger scale, to better manage your appetite. Phase Two is when you'll really start to see the weight drop off.

Phase Three is devoted to transitioning you into the healthy, high-quality diet that's going to allow you to maintain the weight loss you've achieved. You will continue to change what you eat, eliminating more foods that contain empty calories and replacing them with nutritious alternatives. This is your diet for life, and the diet that will give you your best life.

Throughout this book, you will find a lot of information about *why* you will be doing what you're doing. I don't want you to just take the rules I give you at face value; you have a much better chance of sticking to them if you understand both the physiology and the psychology underlying weight loss. With that in mind, I've dedicated the first section of this book to helping you prepare for some of the physical and emotional ups and downs that are an inevitable part of shedding pounds. One of the most difficult aspects of weight loss is facing the prospect that something in your life may be causing you to misuse food and that to stop overeating, you've got to make some changes and, possibly, tough decisions. Being prepared to handle these and other challenges will keep you on track in this program, and if you stay on track, you're going to succeed.

Helping you get ready for change before giving you the tools to do so is one of the things that makes this program different from others. Another is that the Best Life Diet uses physical activity to bolster dietary changes and rewards you for burning more calories. When you're active, you get to eat more, and you'll see that reflected in the eating guidelines I have provided for you.

To reap the benefits of this program, you don't have to engage in structured workouts like taking aerobics classes or even going for brisk walks, but you do need to move your body more in some way. The effect of activity on how many calories you burn goes way beyond the fact that you burn calories while you engage in activity. As I'll explain further in the first and second chapters of this book, there are many different ways being active makes losing weight a hundred times easier. During Phase One, you'll have the opportunity to look at a chart of five different activity levels, find out where you fall on the spectrum now, and then determine which level you feel is within your capacity to reach. Even doing just a little bit more activity will contribute greatly to helping you lose the pounds and keep them off.

OFFERING YOU ONGOING SUPPORT

The Best Life Diet has the ability to evolve to suit your changing needs. I fully expect your eating habits to change as new nutrition information is released and new and improved products come onto the market. But in this fast-paced world, printed material can get dated quickly, so I've developed the website www.thebestlife.com as a companion to this book and program. I'll be using the website to keep you abreast of everything from new, interesting foods (including those bearing the Best Life Diet seal of approval) to research news from the field of nutrition science. The Best Life team will be out there scrutinizing store shelves, checking ingredients, testing recipes, and keeping an ear to the ground to give you frequent updates. There will be articles about eating trends, an exercise library filled with great workouts, techniques for keeping you motivated, tools for self-discovery, and coupons for your favorite healthy foods. This is a diet for life, so the last thing I want is for you to get tired of the foods you're eating or to miss out on news that can benefit your well-being. The world around us changes; the way you eat should change, too.

The website also has the ability to offer you individualized versions of the Best Life Diet with meal plans customized to the specifics you provide, whether you need meal ideas for a low-sodium diet, vegetarian meal plans, or any one of countless other dietary adjustments. You can also sign up for a more structured plan that includes weekly weigh-ins and feedback as well as customized meal plans to make your plan as effective as it can be.

Another feature of www.thebestlife.com is that it can put you in touch with other people who are dealing with the same weight-loss challenges you are. Everyone needs support to succeed at weight loss, and much of that support will come from your friends and family. But acquaintances you meet online can be of great help, too. Hooking you up with others in the program is another way the website can help you well beyond the pages of this book.

LOOKING AT THE WHOLE PICTURE

One thing you'll never hear from me is that making changes in your life is easy. Even making gradual changes, as you will do during this program, can be tough, so I want you to be prepared for the challenge, but also think about the bigger picture and what other rewards you can get from this program besides a slimmer body.

It's not an accident that this program has the word *life* in its name. Losing weight can change your life for the better in ways that far exceed being happier with your appearance. It can even change your life in ways that you would not expect. So many people I've worked with have found that losing weight made them more open to trying new things and going to new places. They became more confident in social situations, too. And all of it—the new people, the new experiences, the new places—resulted in them eventually leading a very different life than before they shed the extra pounds.

The process you go through to lose weight can give you valuable insight into yourself and what it is that's preventing you from having the full life you want. What's more, each step you take toward reaching your weight-loss goal is really a gift that you give yourself. When you eat right and exercise, you are taking care of yourself, treating yourself with respect, and acknowledging that you deserve to be healthy and happy.

The crucial difference between this program and your typical "miracle" diet is that miracle diets tend to give you a big bang—maybe a quick or surprisingly substantial weight loss—that peters out fairly quickly. The beauty of this program is that it provides you with a series of ongoing victories. Each day you take a few small steps, then build on them the day after that. Sure, there may be setbacks—everyone has them—but those victories will add up, and pretty soon you'll be amazed at how different your life has become. And what could be more alluring than the prospect of waking up to your best life? So let's roll up our sleeves and get to work!

UNDERSTANDING YOUR WEIGHT

▶ Right about now, you're probably itching to jump right into this program and see the needle on the scale start inching its way down. If that's the case, I'm happy that you're ready to get going. But it's also important that you be well prepared for the challenges that lie ahead. The process of losing weight can send you on an emotional roller coaster unlike any other, but if you know what's to come, you'll be able to weather the ride. How you handle the inevitable ups and downs can mean the difference between your failure and your success.

This chapter will help prepare you for the changes coming your way. There are two elements of weight loss in particular that can cause frustration and lead people to give up. I want you to understand both of them well so that when the process gets a little rocky you'll know why. This will prevent you from getting discouraged—you'll know that the rocky time is going to pass.

The first challenge you may face is the often erratic nature of weight loss at the beginning of a new program and fluctuating numbers on the scale. When you approach losing weight in the right way—and by that I mean when you increase your activity level, eat regular meals, and consume a nourishing but not overly restrictive diet—you're going to drop pounds, and you're going to drop them in such a way that they're going to stay off. But it might be in a slightly slower and less linear way than you anticipated.

In fact, during the first few weeks of a program of healthful eating—as opposed to a severely restricted one—it's not uncommon for the numbers on the scale to either swing back and forth or move at a snail's pace—or both. If you don't know much about the science behind how your body loses and gains weight, this can be a source of great frustration and even put you in danger of becoming so disappointed that you give up on weight loss altogether (or until the next new diet comes along). But there are good physiological reasons why weight loss can be so fraught with difficulty early in the process. If you hang in there for the long haul, you'll see the results you want; you just need to be ready for all the twists and turns it usually takes to get there.

The second challenge is to discover if there is something in your life that's causing you to misuse food. Many people trying to lose weight look no deeper than the backs of their refrigerators to get at the root of why they eat too much. But being overweight is often a sign that you need to look deep inside *yourself,* not your refrigerator. The real reason you're over-weight may have more to do with fact that something in your life needs to change and less to do with your weakness for French fries. It may be that you're sad or anxious, stressed-out or angry, bored or lonely or feeling out of control—it could be all of them or something else entirely. What's crit-ical is that you find out what in your life is stirring up your emotions and ultimately causing you to turn to food for comfort and distraction. While it's possible to lose weight without giving an iota of attention to your emo-tional life, it's rare—I'd even say impossible—to keep the unaddressed problems from sending you right back into a cycle of losing and regaining weight. People who succeed at reaching their weight-loss goals tend to do some serious soul-searching and, as you stand ready to commit to this pro-gram, it's important that you prepare to do the same.

BODY FAT, WATER RETENTION, AND POUNDS THAT EBB AND FLOW: HOW WEIGHT LOSS WORKS

If you've been following the basic formula for weight loss—consume fewer calories than you burn—for a week or more, it's not unreasonable to ex-pect to see immediate results on the scale. But the way you go about los-ing weight has a significant impact on how much weight you lose in the first weeks of a program. If you go on a restrictive diet and don't exercise, yes, you will see the numbers on the scale plummet. Diets that severely limit calories are designed to help you lose weight fast; that's what draws peo-ple to them—and what draws them back again after they regain the weight. But restrictive diets also provide a false sense of accomplishment because what you lose isn't necessarily body fat, which of course is precisely what you do want to lose. What's more, when you lose weight in this quick-fix way, it almost always comes back (for reasons I'll get to in a minute). You've probably gone on diets that rewarded you with rapid weight loss before and know from experience what I'm talking about.

On the other hand, when you take a more moderate approach that combines diet and exercise, the pounds don't peel off quickly during the first few weeks. That doesn't mean that the diet isn't working. When you learn more about what body weight actually is and how the process of losing it works, you'll be able to take comfort in the fact that you are making progress—even if it doesn't always feel that way in the beginning.

So what *is* going on inside your body? There are many factors that determine how much you weigh, and you'll find a rundown on all of them in the box on page 22. But a lot of what you experience when you start a weight-loss program has to do with the three components that make up your body weight: water, lean tissue, and body fat. Water makes up about *70 percent* of your body weight and is present in the bloodstream, in the digestive tract, and in every cell (including the muscle cells and, to a much lesser degree, the fat cells). Lean tissue refers to a number of different types of cells that make up your muscles, bones, cartilage, hair, and nails. The last component is body fat—fat cells stored mostly in your thighs, hips, backs of the arms, and abdomen, as well as in some less obvious places such as around your vital organs and, sometimes, on the walls of the arteries and veins.

Of the three components of weight, body fat is the one you want to lose, not only because it's what largely determines your size, but also because having too much body fat puts your health at risk. While it may seem like you want to lose water weight, too, it's actually better to hold on to water. I know that may run counter to everything you've ever heard (and desired) about water weight, but there are good reasons for staying well hydrated, which I'll get to shortly.

The first component of body weight I want to talk about is lean tissue. You want to preserve lean tissue—bone, because bone loss weakens your skeleton, increasing your risk of the brittle-bone disease osteoporosis; and muscle, because losing muscle can actually interfere with your ability to burn fat at an optimal rate. Muscle, in fact, plays a vital role in your ability to lose weight. Because muscle is a high-maintenance tissue—meaning that your body must burn quite a few calories to keep it in good working order—it's to your benefit to retain and even gain muscle tissue. It's particularly important that you be aware of this because when you reduce your food intake drastically, the body not only dips into your fat stores for energy (exactly what you *want* to happen), you also lose water, glycogen (a form of carbohydrate stored in your muscles), and even some muscle tissue (exactly what you *don't* want to happen).

Muscle's part in keeping the rate at which you burn calories (your metabolism) running at a significant clip is so important that you want to do everything you can to prevent muscle loss. Even when you're not cutting calories severely—and on this diet you won't be—there are other ways that you can lose muscle tissue. One way is by being inactive; the other is by aging: muscle cells begin to die off through natural attrition as early as your thirties. But, and this is a big but, you won't lose muscle if you use your muscles, which is why increasing your activity level is one of the goals I've set for you in Phase One and why I'll encourage you to keep raising the exercise bar in Phase Two and Phase Three.

Activity not only helps you maintain the muscle you have, it helps in other ways, too. For instance, it can help you build additional muscle so that your metabolism not only doesn't drop, but actually increases. When you exercise regularly, your muscles also increase production of enzymes that allow you to process more oxygen. The more oxygen available, the more calories you're able to burn—this gives your metabolism another significant lift.

The reason I always strongly recommend both cardiovascular and strength-training exercises is because they affect the muscles' impact on calorie burning in different ways. Aerobic exercise promotes the production of the enzymes that boost oxygen consumption and therefore the burning of calories, while strength training is the activity that best helps you maintain and build muscle. It also strengthens the skeleton, helping to stem bone loss and lowering your risk of osteoporosis. Strength training isn't a mandatory part of Phase One, but you can see why I am going to strongly urge you to take it up at some point if you haven't already. It's one of the best ways to spur on the weight-loss process as well as one of the best things you can do to stay vibrant and healthy. You can learn more about strength training, including the most effective strength-training exercises and how do to them correctly, at www.thebestlife.com.

The second of the three components of weight—water—is, I think, the most misunderstood. Water is probably the biggest factor in determining what you weigh in the early weeks of a weight-loss program. If you go about losing weight the wrong way, you will lose a lot of water weight and think that you're having great success. *Don't fall for it!* I can't stress this enough. Losing water creates the illusion that you're losing body fat but will actually *inhibit* your loss of body fat. Here's why.

A primary source of your muscles' fuel is carbohydrates, but in order to store carbohydrate in your muscles, the body must first convert it to a substance called glycogen. And in order to convert carbohydrate to glycogen, you must pair it with water—approximately 2.5 to 3 grams of water per gram of carbohydrate. When you radically reduce the number of calories you take in and in particular the amount of carbohydrates you eat, your body reaches for the carbs stored as glycogen in your muscles. When the glycogen is released, so is the water it was stored with. Your body then eliminates the water and the numbers on the scale go down. Meanwhile, you have lost pounds, but it's primarily pounds of water. What's wrong with that? For one thing, as I've already said, you haven't lost fat. For another, water helps keep your metabolism (and all bodily processes, including fat metabolism) operating properly, ensuring that you burn calories at an efficient rate, which is what is going to help you lose body fat.

The other thing about losing water weight is that as soon as you increase your carbohydrate intake, your muscles will begin retaining water again. That's why many people who thought that they achieved success on a low-carbohydrate diet get thrown for a loop when the numbers on the scale jump back up as soon as they normalize their diet.

It's important to understand that holding on to water is very beneficial both because of how it enhances your ability to burn calories and because your muscles need it to perform well. Whenever you increase your activity, your muscles will store more glycogen, and thus more water, to help them keep up with the demands you're placing on them. You will also add water to your bloodstream, increasing your blood volume and resulting in an increased ability to deliver oxygen, which in turn will increase your capacity to burn more calories.

These changes will cause you to gain, not lose, water weight in the beginning stages of this program, unlike what happens on programs that have a more restricted diet and don't include exercise. I know that this can be disconcerting to some people. When you have increased your activity, are eating more regular meals, and are adhering to an evening cutoff time for food, as you will in Phase One, you'll expect the number on the scale to drop. For many people it will, but for others it may fluctuate and even go up temporarily. And that's not even taking into account the natural water-weight fluctuations you may have to contend with. The amount of water your body retains can easily change depending on what foods you eat (salt and MSG cause water retention, caffeine causes water loss); what nutritional supplements and medications you're taking (your pharmacist or physician should be able to tell you which cause water retention and which cause release); and your hormones (most women retain water each month around the time of their period).

It's critical to remember that the water your body is holding on to because your muscles are using it to store fuel hides the fact that you're losing body fat. Don't be discouraged! Take this water-weight phenomenon in stride. Bear in mind that you want water stored in your muscles and available to keep your metabolism fired up and your muscles operating in high gear so that you don't get fatigued and short yourself on calorie-burning activity. Remember, too, that for most of you, after four to six weeks (and maybe a little longer for others), your initial water-weight gain is going to be behind you.

Because you've probably become accustomed to thinking of water weight as undesirable, you might be upset at the prospect of gaining it. You might even shun exercise because it encourages your muscles to hold on to water. But the additional water you'll be holding on to will help ensure that you lose the right kind of weight—fat! Programs that don't include exercise and diets that dehydrate you through water loss don't help you lose all that much body fat. They only trick you into believing that you're losing fat weight. Going about losing weight the right way is slower and the results you want to see will be longer in coming, but they'll also be longer-lasting.

RECONSIDERING THE SCALE

Weighing yourself too often in the beginning of any program can really wreak havoc with your emotions, because chances are, your weight will go up and down as your body adjusts to your new eating and activity patterns. The frustration that comes from watching these fluctuations causes many people to quit before they see real results. I don't want that to happen to you, so I've developed a very specific weigh-in schedule for each phase of the program. Weigh yourself the first day that you start Phase One, then step off the scale and stay off it for four weeks. No good can come from watching the numbers at this stage—they can be erratic and really are not very relevant to your ultimate results. Plus, there are other ways to gauge your progress. For example, how your clothes fit is a better indicator of what's really going on than the scale. If they fit the same as before you began the Best Life Diet, you've probably lost some body fat; otherwise your clothes would feel tighter because of your water weight gain. If your clothes feel loose, then you've lost even more body fat.

Keep in mind that your body can actually only lose about 3 pounds of body fat a week. This may come as a surprise—so many weight-loss programs promise more (which just goes to show that what they're promising is not just fat loss, but water loss). Since World War II, we have known that there are limits to how much fat the body is willing to part with at a time. This interesting fact was first discovered at the University of Minnesota, where scientists closely studied men who were on semistarvation diets. Much of our basic understanding of weight loss came out of these studies, including the fact that when calories are reduced, the body, in self-preservation, slows the metabolism to reduce calorie burning and fat loss. As a result, even when the calorie reduction is dramatic, the body won't allow a loss of much more than 3 pounds of fat a week.

This research really drives home the point that drastically reducing your calories is destined to backfire. When you drop your calorie intake, it signals your body to conserve as much energy as possible. It doesn't matter that you already have calories stored up in the form of body fat, or that you live where food is abundant: your body still relies on the same mechanisms that helped protect your primitive ancestors in times of famine. Body fat is critical to your survival because it protects your inner organs, insulates you from the cold, and stores vitamins and minerals; your body is going to do all that it can to hang on to a certain amount of it. So ironically, when you eat too little, you're not going to lose as much body fat as you'd expect—and you're certainly not going to lose enough to make suffering through severe deprivation worth the trouble.

Although I'm sure you'd like to lose even more than the 3 pounds of fat per week that your body will allow, that loss can still be pretty unsettling to a system that is naturally inclined to store as much fat as possible. Losing weight at a rate of 1 to 2 pounds per week is a healthier way to go, and that's what you should be looking for on this program. I know that when your expectations are higher, this doesn't sound like much, but now that you know more about what your body is physiologically capable of losing, you should be able to see that dropping 1 to 2 pounds a week is a great accomplishment. I'm not asking you to lower your expectations as much as I'm asking you to take pleasure in each little accomplishment you make.

As you go forward in this program, there may come a time when, although you have passed your initial water-weight gain and have been dropping pounds steadily, it seems as though you've stopped losing weight. This is most likely because your body is reacting to the loss of body fat by adjusting your metabolism to help prevent you from losing more of it. It's similar to what happens when you cut calories drastically; however, if you're still eating a moderate amount of calories and are active, your body will likely readjust. If this weight plateau persists for at least three weeks, then it's an indication that you need to change some things to get your weight loss moving again.

When weight loss stalls for a substantial length of time, it usually means that you've run up against your set point. *Set point* is the level of body fat that your body is preprogrammed to maintain (it's actually a range), and your body will do what it can to keep that level consistent. Everyone has his or her own set point; yours may be entirely different than your skinny next-door neighbor's because your set point is largely determined by genetics. The good news is that activity seems to lower your "fat thermostat" and reset your set point so that you can continue losing. I've seen dozens of clients push past their set point by stepping up their activity level. Making changes in the number of calories you eat can help you push past a plateau as well (although it doesn't pay to reduce your calories too sharply, because then the antistarvation defense mechanism will kick in and slow your weight loss all over again). Once you get beyond the weight ups and downs of Phase One, keeping an eye on the scale will let you know when you've reached your set point and need to make some changes to help you resume dropping pounds.

WHAT DETERMINES YOUR BODY WEIGHT?

Here are seven factors that influence how much you weigh on a purely physiological basis.

1 **Genetics:** Biology is destiny to a certain extent, but don't forget that your parents' lifestyle habits also influenced their weight. Their bodies aren't necessarily exact blueprints for yours.

2 **Food:** What you eat and your calorie intake figure into your weight over time. It takes 3,500 calories to gain a pound, so when you gain weight from overeating, it's generally overeating that has happened over many days, months, or even years.

3 **Medications:** Some medications, including some antidepressants, contraceptives, antipsychotics, and drugs for bipolar disorder and insomnia, may make it harder to lose weight because they alter your metabolism or increase your appetite or both.

4 **Smoking:** Nicotine actually allows your body to stay at a lower weight, as much as 12 to 20 pounds lower, by reducing your set point and dulling hunger. It also gives you something to do with your mouth besides stuff it with food. But smoking simply because you want to weigh less is a terrible idea. In fact, if you smoke, quitting smoking is the single most important health decision you can make. See page 37 for more on smoking.

5 **Involuntary (basal) activity:** Breathing, blinking, pumping your blood—all those involuntary activities you're barely even aware of cost you calories. They help determine your basal metabolic rate.

6 **Basic activity:** You might think of this as nervous energy; it's activities like pacing, jumping up to answer a phone instead of reaching for it, gesturing when you talk, even fidgeting in your chair during a meeting. In the course of a year, all these little moves add up to a big calorie burn-off. In fact, research has shown that thin people tend to do considerably more of this type of activity than heavier folks.

7 **Extra activity:** Anything you do beyond basic activity, whether it's formal exercise, like riding a bike thirty minutes, or just moving, like walking from your car into the grocery store, adds to the amount of calories you burn each day.

ADDRESSING YOUR LIFE—
THE KEY TO YOUR WEIGHT

Some weight-loss programs include a diet and nothing more. Some weight-loss programs team diet and exercise. But few weight-loss programs add a third and, I think, essential ingredient: eliminating emotional eating. You can lose weight by diet alone and you can lose even more weight by combining diet and exercise, but if you're an emotional eater—and most people who struggle with overeating do turn to food to help them cope with some aspect of their lives—you're going to have a hard time keeping that weight off if you don't address the cause of this self-destructive behavior.

When you concentrate on diet and exercise alone, you may be neglecting the issues in your life that caused you to become overweight in the first place; it's like putting a Band-Aid on a wound that needs stitches—a short-term solution that may even allow the problem to worsen. In fact, working on cutting calories and increasing your activity gives you the perfect excuse not to deal with those issues—you've now got other things to worry about, like getting in an hour's walk and packing a healthful lunch. But while you're busy at the gym and in the kitchen, those neglected issues are going to grow until you're not able to ignore them anymore. Then where will you be? Probably right back where you started, misusing food to help you cope with life.

I've seen the consequences of ignoring life issues over and over again—and the happy consequences of addressing them. In my last book, *Total Body Makeover*, I told the stories of people who had successfully lost weight and kept it off. Each person had tried losing weight without confronting any of the emotional reasons they were turning to food, and each of them gained the weight back. It wasn't until they made the effort to find out *why* they always regained the weight, and then made changes in their lives to reduce their need to soothe themselves with food, that they took the weight off for good; they made the decisions it takes to achieve a happier, healthier life. This is, in fact, probably the most important difference between people who are successful at losing weight and maintaining the loss, and people who aren't. To lead the life you've always envisioned for yourself, you may need to make tough choices and perhaps even take a brave leap into the unknown.

One of the goals of the Best Life Diet is to help you do just that. In Phase Two, you'll find guidelines for starting the process of self-discovery, and you'll find additional exercises that will help you take an honest look at your life at www.thebestlife.com. But you can begin the process right here by asking yourself the three questions starting on page 26. The answers may show you where your life is out of balance.

The imbalance could be caused by one of a hundred things. In consulting and meeting with many people about their weight, I've found that the problems that lead to overeating are as varied as the people who suffer from them. Maybe you're dissatisfied with your career, or it's causing you more stress than you can handle. Maybe you're in a relationship with someone who's making you unhappy. Maybe you're not in a relationship with someone and *that's* making you unhappy. Maybe the experiences you had as a child have made you severely insecure as an adult, so that even though you've achieved professional and financial success, deep down you feel like a fraud and eat out of guilt and shame. Maybe you've never achieved the professional and financial success you hoped for and the pressure of not having enough money is driving you to the refrigerator. Maybe you're actually very happy with your life but you grew up associating food with celebration and now it's gotten out of control. Whatever it is, you're the only person who can pinpoint the problem. And ultimately, you're also the only person who can make the decision to resolve it.

I'm not going to tell you that making big life changes is easy. The truth is that it's usually the most demanding part of weight loss. Most people think the toughest thing about losing weight is getting to the gym and giving up foods they like. But all that is easy when you compare it to making significant changes in your life. Change almost always involves difficult choices, maybe even as difficult as leaving a job or a relationship, confronting a family member, severing a friendship, or altering something fundamental about yourself, such as the way you relate to other people. It takes courage to tackle these types of changes, but it may be absolutely necessary if you hope to achieve long-term weight loss.

Look at it this way: if you're like most people, you're probably trying to lose weight so that you look better and feel better about yourself—that is, you want to be happy. But weight loss alone cannot make you happy. Sure, losing weight will boost your confidence and self-esteem for a short time, but real joy is only going to come to you if you clear up the issues in your life that send you running to the refrigerator. Being a thinner person isn't going to remedy the relationship you have with your significant other or make your job less stressful or sow the seeds of family harmony. These are things that won't change if you sweep them under the rug while you work on sculpting your muscles and paring down your calories; they'll only change when you give them the attention they deserve. Do that and you'll improve *all* aspects of your life, make the weight-loss process easier, and ensure that the results are permanent. Weight loss will come—it'll just be the icing on the cake.

ASK YOURSELF THE TOUGH QUESTIONS

When was the last time you really took the time to think about who you are, what you want, and why you really want it? Life these days is so busy, so packed with commitments, responsibilities, and an onslaught of information to keep up with that it's rare for anyone to sit down and get to know him- or herself better. If that's true for you, then there's a good chance that you're operating on autopilot, making decisions and taking on challenges without really understanding what you truly want and need from life.

The purpose of the following three questions is to help you give some serious thought to one thing: yourself. I want you to explore what's happening in your life now, examine your motives, and replay events of the past so that you can enter into this program with a better knowledge of what's going to help you succeed. If you're an emotional eater, I suspect that you probably already know the reasons why you misuse food, but if you've dropped and regained pounds many times over, it's an indication that you're not facing up to those issues, or not making the tough choices you need to. These questions may give you an opportunity to see yourself plainly and without judging yourself. The point of this exercise isn't to label your behavior "bad" or shame you for not taking action in certain areas of your life. It's simply to help you find out if something needs to change so that you can get on with the business of changing it.

I encourage you to write down your answers to these questions. When you're just sitting around mulling a question over, it's easy for your mind to wander. Make your responses more formal and you'll be less likely to get distracted. You might even be surprised by what gets put on paper once your pen starts moving.

1. WHY ARE YOU OVERWEIGHT?

I've asked this question of many people, and here are some of the answers I've heard: "I have to eat out a lot for business," "My husband isn't support-ive," "I have to keep sweets in the house for my family and I can't resist them," "I just haven't found the right diet," "I have a desk job," "My fam-ily commitments are my first priority," "Healthy food is too expensive," "The holidays always trip me up," "I don't like to sweat," "I don't have time to exercise." These predicaments may all be challenges to the weight-loss process, but they're not real reasons why someone is overweight. These re-sponses are simply justifications, or what I like to call "surface responses." Surface responses are an attempt to take the pressure off yourself and lay the blame somewhere else. If you have a surface response to this question, you're letting yourself off the hook.

What I want to hear from you instead are the authentic feelings and reactions that lead you to overeat. If you sit down on the couch with a car-ton of ice cream after the kids have gone to bed, it's not because your kids demand that you have ice cream in the house, but it may be because you're so worn out by the kids that you feel you have to reward yourself with some-thing. Or maybe it's because you have a meeting with your boss the follow-ing day and ice cream helps keep your anxiety at bay. Maybe it's because you and your spouse fought about putting the kids to bed and ice cream soothes your anger. Maybe it's because you don't feel as though your fam-ily appreciates you. *Why,* in other words, are you eating? What is the deeper, *real* reason, not the superficial one?

Do you sit at a desk most of the day? Lots of people have seden-tary jobs and still find a way to exercise. Maybe you feel depressed about something—a relationship, the stagnant state of your career—and don't feel like you have the energy or desire to exercise. Maybe you have trou-ble committing to things, exercise being just one of many activities that you start but always end up dropping.

In order to benefit from this process, you need to be ready to be truly honest with yourself. In doing so, you're saying, "I really want to change," and that opens the door to making that wish a reality.

I understand why many people are reluctant to admit their personal weaknesses. There's nothing that can make you feel as vulnerable. And once you admit you need to change something, there's the realization that you, and only you, can change it. That's scary, because what if you can't? I'm here to tell you that you can. You absolutely can, no matter what it is that you wish to change. One woman I worked with was very insecure about her professional capabilities, and to compensate she became very confrontational with everyone at work. As a consequence, she had poor relationships with all her colleagues. Her unhappiness at work was eating away at her—and she was eating everything in sight to make up for it. Before she could ever really take off the weight she'd gained, she was going to have to shore up her self-esteem, alter her behavior, and mend some fences.

Getting over your fear of the truth and admitting what about your life needs to change is what's going to set you on the path to change and ultimately set you free. The more honest and open you are, the closer it's going to bring you to a resolution. Virtually everybody who's overweight reaches a point where they look in the mirror or step on the scale and find that they've reached a weight they can no longer abide—they don't want to have that body anymore, and they set out to change it. I want you to have that same experience, not only with your weight, but in all the areas of your life that are out of kilter. Decide that you're not going to take it anymore and work on changing what needs to be changed. That's what's going to lead to weight loss and, more important, *your* best life.

2. WHY DO YOU WANT TO LOSE WEIGHT?

This is a question I ask clients when we first start our work together. If someone answers simply, "I want to look better," I consider it another surface response and I encourage him or her to dig deeper. This process needs to start with you above all being truthful with yourself about why you want to lose weight. If the first thing that comes to mind is that you want to look better, well, *why* do you want to look better? Is it because you don't feel that the way you look is acceptable to other people? If so, you may need to look closer at your relationships. Maybe you're afraid that your significant other will leave you for someone better-looking. Well, what does that say about the relationship between the two of you? Is your weight or the relationship itself the real problem? Maybe you want people at work to take you more seriously, but what's going on with your professional life that's making you reflect on your personal habits? Maybe you feel lonely and think it's hard to attract someone because you're overweight. Whether that's true or not, it also signals that you may need to make other changes in your life that will enable you to meet the right person. (Look around you—it's not only thin people who have partners.)

In pursuing weight loss, most people are pursuing happiness. It's important, though, to think about *how* exactly you see weight loss bringing you happiness. Can becoming thinner really make all the other worries in your life go away? I get concerned whenever someone ties weight loss to happiness, because there are only two possible outcomes. Either you never reach the size you're hoping for and you're not happy, or you do lose the weight only to find that it doesn't make you happy. Where does that leave you? It almost always leads to the misuse of food and back to being overweight. To me, this kind of thinking is turned around. Losing weight isn't the key to happiness—happiness is the key to losing weight. On page 85, I'm going to introduce you to an exercise called the Circle of Life. I've included details about this exercise in past books, and it's one of the exercises you'll find in more detail on www.thebestlife.com. The Circle of Life can help you to see where the *real* potential source of your happiness lies. When you tap that source, you're not going to have to turn to food for comfort anymore.

I'm not saying that losing weight alone can't bring you some degree of happiness or help you feel better about yourself. It can. But don't put all your eggs in one emotional basket. Take the focus off how losing weight is going to make you look and put it on how losing weight can help you improve your life. To me, one of the best reasons for wanting to lose weight is a desire to take control of and enhance all aspects of your life. Once, when I asked a client what his motivation for trying to lose weight was, he told me, "I'm just so sick of the way I behave." I saw it as a good sign that he was making the connection between his actions and their consequences and that what he really wanted to change was the way he lived his life. He had set a bigger, more ambitious, and, I'd venture to say, more important goal than simply wanting to look good. I'm asking you to do likewise. Don't settle for just aiming to look better; shift your priorities and set your sights on a better life—the life you deserve.

3. WHY HAVE YOU BEEN UNABLE
TO MAINTAIN WEIGHT LOSS IN THE PAST?

I had one client who had trouble coming up with a reason why she'd always regain the weight she lost. But after thinking about it for a while, she remembered that when she was younger, her mother would always discourage her attempts to lose weight by saying, "The way you eat? You're not going to do it." That was quite some time ago, but my client still had her mother's prediction of failure in the back of her mind.

Family members and friends often say things that can have a negative effect when sometimes all they are really trying to do is help. I think we're particularly sensitive to things our parents or those close to us say; it's easy to take things the wrong way. But right or wrong, if you think that someone close to you doesn't believe in you, it can adversely affect your view of yourself. And if you don't believe in your ability to lose weight, you probably won't achieve weight-loss success. Many people have a core belief that they're not meant to be happy or deserve happiness: they'd rather have their beliefs confirmed than achieve true happiness, and so they find ways to sabotage themselves.

Take the time to think back on what has caused you to fail in the past; it's another opportunity to take a close look at your attitudes and your actions and the relationship between the two. If you've ever progressed far on a weight-loss program only to revert to your old habits and gain all of the pounds back, replay what went on in your mind. What was the trigger that turned you from someone who was eating healthfully to someone whose eating was out of control? If you can discover what it is, you'll have a good clue about what in your life is driving you to eat. Being honest about what's wrong with your life shows that you're ready to start the healing process. It's also quite possible that your attempt to lose weight was thwarted by an eating and exercise plan that was too rigorous, or maybe not rigorous enough. (This program is going to remedy that by providing you with a realistic plan for improving your eating and exercise habits.)

TAKING STEPS TO CHANGE YOUR LIFE

Answering the questions in the previous section is just the first step that will help you change any self-destructive habits. In *Total Body Makeover,* I devoted a great deal of space to the four defining principles that I believe lead to success in any endeavor, including weight loss. Truthfulness is one of them. It's crucial to take the blinders off and see who you really are, why you do the things you do, and what's really going on in your life. Admit your weaknesses and do what you need to do to change them.

The other three principles are responsibility, commitment, and inner strength. Taking responsibility means that you stop being a victim and laying the blame for the things you don't like about your life on someone or something else. And that goes for things both past and present. Life isn't free of challenges and adversity, and maybe you have had more than your fair share; but *how* you react to events is within your control. Taking responsibility means being willing to take the reins of change. It's only going to happen if *you* make it happen.

There are probably many things in your life you're committed to: your friends, your family, your job. Now, however, is the time to commit to yourself. Act as if you're signing a contract with yourself (in previous books, I've actually included a "Contract with Myself" for readers to sign, and you can find one now on www.thebestlife.com). In other words, take your commitment seriously and don't let yourself down.

The challenges that lie ahead of you require inner strength. People who employ that strength (everybody has it, but only some people choose to use it) don't go out into the world thinking that everything is going to be easy. On the contrary, they acknowledge that to get what they want in life they're going to face some difficult times, but they will get through them. Inner strength, willpower, self-discipline, resolve—whatever you want to call it, it's there deep inside you. When you take a proactive approach to improving your life, it's going to boost your self-esteem, and the better you feel about yourself, the more motivated you're going to feel and, ultimately, the more successful at achieving your goals you're going to be.

Practicing the principles of honesty, responsibility, commitment, and inner strength are going to help you with every aspect of this program, including coming to grips with emotional eating. Eliminating emotional eating is a progression; it doesn't happen overnight. The length of time it takes to mend what's broken in your life, however, is not all that important. What is important is that you keep working toward your goals and that you derive satisfaction from each small step you take in that direction. People who are successful at achieving their best life don't wait for their lives to be perfect in order to feel satisfied; they find it in the pursuit of happiness. They get gratification from each move they make toward building a beautiful life for themselves—as should you, because every step is truly a thrilling accomplishment. If you can become less concerned with achieving big, exciting results, you're going to get more satisfaction and enjoyment from the process of change. And that, ironically, is going to help you get, yes, big, exciting results.

PHASE ONE

▶ When you look at the following box that lists your objectives for Phase One, you'll probably be surprised: There's almost nothing in there about changing what or how much you eat. Instead, the primary goals of this phase are to change the way you organize your meals and to increase your activity level. I want you to add a healthy breakfast to your day, but you don't have to worry about adding or subtracting foods from your diet at this point.

Whenever I tell clients who are trying to lose weight that I don't want them to change what or how much they're eating, I always face some resistance. They're *ready* to change what they eat, and they're ready to change it *now*! They want to clean up their diet and stop overeating. I completely understand the urge to get going and to see some quick results, but my approach is different. Everything you do during the next four weeks (and perhaps a little longer) is going to enhance the weight-loss results you get in Phase Two, the phase devoted to taking off the majority of the pounds you

PHASE ONE

TIME FRAME: A minimum of four weeks

WEIGH IN: Weigh to get your starting weight; then no weighing in for at least four weeks

FOCUS: Moving more and changing your meal patterns

OBJECTIVES:

▶ Increase your activity level

▶ Stop eating at least two hours before bedtime

▶ Eat three meals, including a nutritious breakfast, plus at least one snack daily

▶ Stay hydrated

▶ Eliminate alcohol, for now

▶ Bolster your diet with daily supplements

JUDGING YOUR SUCCESS: Check in at week four to see whether you're ready to move on need to lose. But more than that, Phase One will get you comfortable with some healthy habits that will ensure that you keep the pounds off for good.

Most diets start you off by having you substantially reduce your calories. That initial weight loss may seem great, but what it really does is give you a false sense of success. As I talked about at length in "Understanding Your Weight," when you quickly drop a lot of pounds at the beginning of a diet, you're typically not losing all that much body fat; you're losing a lot of water weight. A steep reduction in calories also triggers your body's starvation defense mechanisms, so it ultimately slows the weight-loss process down. It makes you hungrier, too, and leads to feelings of deprivation that can cause you to go back to your old habits. So while a fast-and-furious approach to weight loss is very seductive, you'll be much better off if you don't fall for the seduction of a quick fix.

In Phase One, you're going to increase your activity level so that your metabolism is operating in high gear when you begin cutting calories more vigorously; that's going to keep the starvation effect from kicking in. You're also going to be changing your meal patterns, which will also help you maximize your calorie burning and keep your appetite in check. When you eat regular meals and snacks and have an eating cutoff time (all practices you'll be establishing during this phase), you won't have hunger highs and lows, and that's going to help you deal with the calorie cutting you'll be initiating in subsequent phases.

There are also some other healthy practices you're going to establish during this phase. First and foremost, if you smoke, I'm going to recommend that you quit before you go any further in the program. This is the absolute best investment you can make for your well-being.

During this phase, you'll also eliminate alcohol, with the option to put it back into your diet in Phase Three. Drinking alcohol makes it harder to lose weight for several reasons, and avoiding it for a time will remove all of the obstacles it can put in your path. During this phase, you'll also begin drinking more water, another healthy habit that will help prime your body for weight loss. For nutritional insurance, I'm going to have you take a good multivitamin and mineral supplement, and I strongly recommend that you take an omega-3 fatty acid supplement and, if needed, a calcium supplement daily. You'll be adding a healthy breakfast to your day during this phase as well, but other than that, the kinds of foods you eat and how much of them you eat at each sitting can stay the same.

Incorporating these simple changes is going to get your metabolism revved up and your body primed for losing weight, just like a car that's idling and ready to hit the road. Phase One is all about making positive investments in yourself so you're able to accomplish consistent weight loss and so the challenges you'll be facing later on in Phases Two and Three (that's when you'll be making significant changes to what you eat) are much easier.

And you will be rewarded with other immediate benefits. Just restructuring your meals will most likely lower your calorie intake and, depending on what your eating habits are like now, maybe even significantly. I've had many clients who've reached their goal weight just by meeting the objectives in Phase One, especially when they significantly increase their level of activity. You may or may not be as lucky. I hope you are, though bear in mind that not everyone achieves the same results, just as not everyone has the same amount of weight to lose (or the same habits to break). But whatever the immediate outcome, the investments you make during Phase One are extremely important and are going to have a big impact on your success down the road.

The ultimate goal of this program is to help you adopt a way of life and establish habits that contribute to both weight loss and your overall well-being. During Phase One, you're investing in yourself in order to attain that goal. That doesn't mean you have to be perfect, but it does mean you have to be purposeful about how you live. You need to recast yourself as someone who, to the best of his or her ability, lives consciously. And it all begins right here.

TIME FRAME

You should stay in Phase One for a minimum of four weeks; however, at the end of four weeks, I'll give you some guidelines (see page 68) to help you assess whether you should move on to the next phase or not. If you're losing weight at a healthy pace, I'm going to encourage you to ride out your success in Phase One for a while longer. If not, you can move on to Phase Two, the primary weight-loss stage of this program.

WEIGH IN

Before you go any further, step on the scale to get your starting weight. Then put the scale away, and don't look at it for another four weeks. I know the temptation to weigh yourself regularly will be great, but DON'T DO IT! Fluctuations in your weight at this early stage (and for most people there *will* be fluctuations) can really send you on an emotional roller coaster. I want you to avoid that inner turmoil, especially because the scale really isn't a good indicator of what's going on in your body at this point.

As you might remember from the previous chapter, the numbers on the scale don't adequately reflect fat loss, due to the water-weight gain that generally accompanies increases in physical activity. So during this initial period, forget about the scale; instead, practice patience and give your new, healthier habits time to work. If you're always watching the scale and worrying about the numbers, it's going to be harder to stay the course.

Besides, you won't really need the scale at this point to know if you're losing weight. When you do shed pounds in this phase, you're going to know it by how your clothes feel. At this stage, that's the best indicator of how well you're doing. If your clothes hug your body similar to the way they did when you first started, it's a sign that you're losing some body fat; it's just being replaced by water weight. You'll know that you're losing a good bit of body fat if your clothes feel loose; that's a really good sign in Phase One.

A QUICK WORD ABOUT SMOKING

I'll say it again: If you smoke, kicking the cigarette habit is the absolute best investment you can make for yourself right now, at the outset of this program. Quitting smoking and trying to lose weight may seem to work against each other, and in some ways they do. The nicotine in cigarettes keeps your metabolism elevated, so when you smoke, you not only burn more calories, but your body also settles in at a lower weight. But what a price to pay for staying slimmer! Smoking is the number one preventable cause of death; I can't think of anything that predisposes you to so many kinds of disease as readily as smoking.

And, if you think about it, despite the metabolic boost, you may not really be getting that much of a calorie-burning advantage from smoking if it keeps you from exercising at a vigorous pace. Most smokers find it difficult to work out effectively because their lungs are so congested and the oxygen-carrying capacity of their blood is so diminished. If you become a non-smoker, you can exercise with greater ease and get a much more powerful calorie-burning advantage. But the real issue here, of course, is your health.

It may not seem like a good time to quit smoking, because this program is going to give you plenty of other things to concentrate on and you may feel like the last thing you want to deal with now is nicotine withdrawal. If you don't think you can handle all the changes at once, I would recommend that you delay working on your diet and work on stopping smoking first. This program is about attaining your best life, and that means your healthiest life, so it really doesn't make sense to get going if you haven't put your number one health concern behind you first.

Plus, some of the changes you'll be making during the Best Life Diet will actually make quitting smoking easier. Exercise, for instance, helps improve your mood, so you may feel less of a need to smoke (the time you spend working out will fill some of the time you used to spend puffing away, too). And if you have the right mind-set, changing your diet and quitting smoking at the same time won't make you feel overburdened but, rather, highly motivated.

Although it may seem like it would be easier to quit smoking *after* you lose weight, in most cases, that's a mistake. Once you've already lost weight, fear of putting it back on and undermining all your hard work may weaken your resolve to quit. If you do decide to quit after you've already lost weight, you probably will put some of the weight back on, and that can be discouraging—maybe even discouraging enough to make you pick up the habit again or gain back all of the weight you lost. Either way, waiting is risky. *Now* is the perfect time to quit smoking. You can find more about the effects of smoking and ways to kick the habit at www.thebestlife.com.

PHASE ONE OBJECTIVES

Increase Your Activity

While it's possible to lose weight and keep it off without being active, it's very difficult—so difficult that not many people are ever really able to do it. One of the main benefits of activity is that it counters some of the negative effects of calorie reduction by helping to preserve muscle and prevent the body's natural inclination to slow your metabolism when faced with consuming less food. You'll learn more about both of these processes later in this section, but let's just say for now that there's a good reason why the people who are most successful at losing and maintaining weight loss do so through a combination of diet and exercise.

Experts in the weight-loss field have always maintained that pairing diet and exercise is the best approach to shedding pounds, and in the last few years, an ongoing project called the National Weight Control Registry (NWCR) has confirmed it. The NWCR is devoted to looking at what separates people who successfully lose weight and keep it off from those who fail. Directed by researchers from Brown Medical School and the University of Colorado, the registry has so far tracked more than five thousand people who've lost at least thirty pounds and kept them off for more than a year. This project spawned several different studies that have investigated the realities of weight loss, including a study that looked at how one particular group of people lost weight and kept the pounds from piling back on. What the researchers found was that even though some members of the group followed a formal weight-loss program while others lost weight by their own devices, all of them succeeded because of a combination of diet and exercise. There may be many recipes for weight loss, but as this study shows, activity is a critical ingredient.

If you haven't already incorporated activity into your life, I really urge you to do so now. If you used to exercise and now you're on a sort of hiatus—maybe you had a baby and never returned to your regular workouts, or you got super busy at work and let your gym membership lapse— you already know how great exercise can make you feel. Take this opportunity to get back on track. If you're already active, I hope you'll bump it up at least a level as part of your commitment to this program.

There are so many reasons to be active, including the fact that it is one of the best things you can do for your health. I could bore you with the details of how being active lowers the risk of almost every disease imaginable (from most types of cancer to diabetes to osteoporosis) and how it can significantly improve your quality of life (by improving mood, helping you to sleep better, keeping your mind sharp, reducing your susceptibility to colds and flu, and, yes, improving your sex life). But I think you've heard all of that before, and it's either motivated you to exercise or not. So let me get to what I think may convince you to increase the amount of activity you're presently doing: the more you move your body, the easier losing weight on this—or any—weight-loss program is going to be.

Cutting calories can be challenging, so the fewer calories you have to eliminate from your diet, the better. This is where activity comes in. Exercise increases the number of calories you burn (in more ways than you may think), and that means you can eat more and still achieve the negative energy balance you need to lose weight. (Being able to eat more also increases the chances that you'll get all the nutrients you need.) When you're trying to cut back on the amount of food you eat, those extra calories can really feel like a windfall. And on this program, they really are a windfall because the more activity you incorporate into your day, the more Anything Goes calories you'll get. These extra calories, which you'll learn how to tally on page 119 and can begin using in Phase Three, can be "spent" each day or week on your favorite foods. So you see, activity really does make the whole weight-loss process easier: if you move more, you can eat more, and if you can eat more, you'll be less stressed-out about feeling deprived.

I want to add that if you break out of activity levels 0 and 1 and move up to Level 2 or higher, the rewards are particularly sweet. (See the Best Life Activity Scale, starting on page 44.) When you work out regularly, you'll open up a whole new world of food to yourself, not only because you're burning more calories, but also because you need food to keep your muscles properly fueled. Research shows that there's a nice window of opportunity in the thirty minutes right after exercising to replenish your muscles with carbohydrates and protein. In this post-activity state, muscles act like sponges and absorb nutrients at a particularly high rate, so it's actually to your benefit to have a snack, such as a sweet yogurt shake, an energy or granola bar, some low-fat chocolate milk, a handful of chocolate-covered peanuts, some low-fat pudding, even a homemade milkshake made with one cup of skim milk and a heaping half cup of light ice cream. You don't have to feel guilty for eating something delicious, because you've earned it.

Of course, this is not the only perk of exercise. Increasing your activity is going to make you feel more energetic, improve your mood, and boost your confidence in your own capabilities. Each of these things will contribute to your weight-loss efforts. With more energy, you'll move more as you go about your daily routine, burning a greater number of calories throughout your day as a result. When your mood is improved, you'll have less of a need to turn to food for emotional support, and the increased confidence you get from being an active person will also help motivate you to stay on this program. I know so many people who've overhauled their eating habits without prompting after becoming active. They simply fell in love with how strong and healthy physical activity made them feel, and they wanted to enhance the process by eating more nutritiously.

If you already exercise, you're getting some of these great benefits right now. However, the fact that you want to drop some weight despite being active means that you probably need to raise the bar a bit higher. If you fall on the opposite side of the spectrum and aren't very active (or aren't active at all), the rewards I just mentioned are in your future. All it's going to take is a very moderate increase each day in how much you move your body. It doesn't even have to be formal exercise; it can be that you just walk a couple thousand steps more each day. As long as you move more, you're going to benefit. And once you do, you may find that you're inspired to move up another level, then another, and maybe even another. The healthier and more fit you become, the more comfortable you're going to feel exercising.

The rate at which you burn calories is a strong determinant of how much you weigh, so I think it's important that you get a sense of what actually happens to your metabolism when you exercise. That information is followed by the Best Life Activity Scale, which will help you determine how much you're moving your body right now and how much more you're willing to move it.

No matter where you are on the scale (unless of course you're at the very top), I want you to move up a level, but I also want you to select a goal that's within your ability to reach, not just for a few weeks but forever. Don't commit to an exercise program that you won't be able to stick with because once you start failing to meet the goals you've set out for yourself, you're going to feel guilty and defeated. What will inevitably happen then is that those feelings will discourage you from holding on to all the other healthy changes you're making with this program. So make room in your life for as much activity as you can reasonably handle right now, then periodically revisit the question "Can I do more?" as you begin each new phase of the Best Life Diet and every few months after that on an ongoing basis.

THE WEIGHT-LOSS EDGE
ONLY ACTIVITY CAN GIVE YOU

I'm sure you're very familiar with the fact that activity burns calories. Every time you move, whether you're taking a brisk forty-five-minute walk around your neighborhood, huffing away on an elliptical trainer for thirty minutes, strolling around the grocery store, or bending down to pick up laundry, you burn calories in varying amounts. This is what most people think about when they think about the energy-expenditure payoff of activity, yet it really is only one of several different ways that activity helps you burn more calories.

Activity, for instance, actually has an "afterburn" effect—that is, it can raise your metabolism for hours after you've stopped exercising. Once you step off the treadmill, stop digging in your garden, or return home from a walk in the park, the rate at which you burn calories remains higher than normal. It doesn't remain at the same rate as when you're, say, jogging or walking, but it stays higher than usual and doesn't slow back down for quite some time. In this sense, you may think of activity as the gift that keeps on giving—kind of like money in a savings account. If you put a nice chunk of change in the bank, a pretty great thing to begin with, then you earn interest on top of that without even lifting a finger. Likewise, you burn a good chunk of calories while exercising; then you get the bonus of burning more calories without any extra effort. It seems like a really good deal to me.

You get this post-exercise metabolism boost whenever you do any type of activity, whether it's aerobic exercise (which gets your heart rate up and accelerates your breathing), strength training with weights or bands, or other activities such as calisthenics, Pilates, or yoga. Some research has shown that one's metabolism can stay elevated for up to sixteen hours after exercise. Not surprisingly, the more vigorous your exercise, the longer the afterburn effect; however, even little bursts of activity, like walking up a few flights of stairs, can give your metabolism a small extended lift.

Activity also affects your metabolism by influencing the amount of muscle you have. Muscle is a very hungry tissue. It takes quite a few calories just for the body to maintain it, and the more muscle you have, the more calories you burn, even when you're just sitting around doing nothing. But muscle deteriorates naturally with age if you don't do anything to prevent it. Drastically cutting calories also puts muscle tissue at risk because when you eat less food, your body doesn't just turn to your fat stores for fuel but also feeds on your muscles.

Because muscle and metabolism are so intimately related, it's important that, at the very least, you keep the muscle tissue you have intact to prevent any slowdown in the rate at which you burn calories. It's even better if you can build additional muscle, because that will raise your metabolism. Strength training is the best type of exercise for maintaining and adding muscle, but aerobic exercise helps your muscles burn calories at a higher rate by promoting an increase in enzymes that make your muscles more metabolically active. If you want to ensure that your body is burning calories at its maximum capacity, then including both aerobic exercise and strength training in your regimen is the ultimate way to go.

There is also one more weight-loss-related benefit of activity I want to address, and that's the relationship between physical activity and your set point. When you exercise, scores of physiological changes take place; activity literally alters the chemistry of your body. One of those changes is that your set point—the level of body fat that your body is programmed to maintain—drops. In other words, your body will carry less fat. Usually, if you significantly decrease the number of calories you eat, your metabolism will slow down. This is the body's defense mechanism to prevent starvation. This may seem crazy, since you're probably far from starving, but this antistarvation set point—defending mechanism was passed down from your ancestors who lived in a time when rapid weight loss usually signaled something dire, such as famine. Times, of course, have evolved, but the set point reflex hasn't.

When you exercise, the extra activity resets your "fat thermostat" so when you try to drop pounds, your body doesn't put up a big fight by slow-ing your metabolism to a crawl. Instead, it allows you to lose more body fat than you would otherwise. You may still eventually hit a plateau at which you run up against your new set point; however, increasing your activity slightly once more can help you push past it again.

So let's recap: activity burns calories, allowing you to eat more food while still shedding pounds. It revs up your metabolism, increasing your energy expenditure above and beyond your normal capacity. It prevents the loss of muscle tissue, thereby counteracting an age- and/or calorie-cutting-related metabolic slowdown, and it lowers your fat thermostat. Could there possibly be a reason *not* to be active? I rest my case.

ESTABLISHING YOUR ACTIVITY LEVEL

Everybody moves. What I want to help you do is move a little, preferably even a lot, more. First, though, you need to establish your starting point by locating your level of activity on the Best Life Activity Scale. Just like jumping on the scale at the outset of this phase gave you a weight benchmark, finding your activity level will give you a point of reference for exercise. I recommend, however, that you read *all* of the levels and not stop reading once you find the category you fall into. That way you can get an idea of not only where you are on the continuum now, but also where you want to ultimately (and can realistically) go, both in the immediate future and further down the road.

The Best Life Activity Scale

The Best Life Activity Scale is composed of six different levels of physical activity. Each level includes an aerobic component and a steps-per-day component. You don't need to monitor your aerobic exercise *and* monitor your steps per day; the two are interchangeable and simply refer to different ways of calculating how much you're moving. Aerobic exercise is gauged in minutes per week; steps per day is, as you would expect, gauged by the number of steps you take per day. That number should include all the steps you take while just going about your daily activities *and* any steps you take while doing formal exercise such as brisk walking or jogging. To

SOME OTHER WEIGHT-RELATED PERKS FROM EXERCISE (YES, THERE'S MORE!)

▶ **More everyday energy.** People who exercise regularly seem to attack life with more vigor. They simply have more energy. They move more and they move faster throughout the day, and as a result they burn a greater number of calories without even trying. If you're unfit, physical activity can make you feel more fatigued than usual. But after a few weeks, being active gives you renewed and enhanced vitality, and that translates into more everyday movement: jumping up to answer the door instead of just saying "come in"; getting up to get something from your bedroom instead of asking one of your kids to bring it to you; pacing while you talk on the phone instead of sitting. Over the course of a day, all of those little moves add up to a significant increase in energy expenditure. In the course of a year, that can add up to substantial weight loss.

▶ **Reduced appetite.** One other benefit of physical activity is that it often helps you tame your appetite. You may get a little hungrier if you exercise than if you don't (especially when you're just beginning an exercise regimen or are in the process of bumping it up a level), but not enough to compensate for the calories you'll burn through activity. You'll still end up taking in less energy than you expend, causing weight to drop off.

One additional explanation for activity's effect on appetite may be that when you get in shape, you'll feel motivated not to undo your hard work by overeating. You'll be more attuned to your body and more mindful of how much food (and what kind) you're taking in. Another possible explanation has to do with brain chemistry. I'll talk more about this in the next chapter, but to state it briefly, some research suggests that people who overeat tend to have a lack of receptors for brain chemicals that make us feel pleasure, which is why they keep eating: it simply takes more food to get the same satisfaction signals that other people get with less. But scientists have also shown that exercise can increase the number of pleasure receptors in the brain. So even if you have a physiological disadvantage that makes you prone to overeat, exercise can help you overcome it, reducing your need to pile your plate too high.

determine your steps per day, you'll need a pedometer, a clip-on counting device that you can wear all day. (Sportline makes a number of great models.) You can purchase one at most sporting goods stores or on www.thebestlife.com.

Neither steps per day or aerobic activity is interchangeable with strength training, which is part of levels 3, 4, and 5. If you are at one of those levels, calculate how much strength training you do separately.

Level 0 You're at Level 0 when any activity you do beyond what it takes to get through your day is purely accidental. Physical activity just isn't on your radar. In fact, you move only when you have to, and because of the way you've set up your life, that's not very often. You only take the stairs when the elevator is out of order, and anytime friends or family ask you to go for a walk, you find a convenient excuse to turn them down (wrong shoes, knee hurts, other commitments). You drive everywhere, maybe have a desk job, and usually just hang around on the couch at night, so your daily movement is minimal, which, you have to admit, is how you like it.

> **AEROBIC EXERCISE:** none
> *or*
> **STEPS PER DAY:** 3,499 or less
> **STRENGTH TRAINING:** none

Level 1 You're at Level 1 if you see the value in activity, so you try to move as much as you can. You may have a job that keeps you on your feet— maybe you're a nurse, waitress, landscaper, or teacher—or perhaps you just make an extra effort to move throughout the day. Maybe you often go for a stroll after dinner or ride bikes with your kids. At work, you'll walk to a colleague's office instead of using email, take the stairs when you can, and return your shopping cart to the front of the store instead of leaving it next to your car, just so you can get a few more steps in. Maybe you get off a stop or two early when you're taking public transportation and walk the rest of the way. You may be someone who hasn't participated in structured exercise since high school. Or maybe you used to have a regular workout program, but some change in your life such as having kids or sustaining an injury led you to quit, and you haven't picked it up again. In general, you look for creative ways to move more throughout the day.

> **LIGHT AEROBIC EXERCISE:** 60–90 minutes per week
> *or*
> **STEPS PER DAY:** approximately 3,500–5,999
> **STRENGTH TRAINING:** none

Level 2 You're at Level 2 if you have a structured and consistent exercise schedule. It's fairly moderate, but it's helped you reap some cardiovascular, body-shaping, and calorie-burning benefits. You may work out any number of ways—by yourself on a stationary bike, in a kickboxing class at a gym, at home with an aerobics DVD, or with a fellow walker on the streets of your neighborhood—but you always get in at least three thirty-minute sessions a week.

> AEROBIC EXERCISE: 3 times a week, at least 90–150 minutes per week
> *or*
> STEPS PER DAY: approximately 6,000–9,999
> STRENGTH TRAINING: none

Level 3 You're at Level 3 if you're serious about exercise and work out at least five and possibly six days a week. On at least four of those days, you do cardiovascular exercise—usually the same workout, whether it be walking, jogging, swimming, or something like going to a spinning or aerobic dance class—for a total of at least 150 minutes a week. At least two days a week, you strength-train with weights, performing at least six different exercises per session. You're so committed to activity that on the weekends, you also take leisurely but long walks.

> AEROBIC EXERCISE: 5 times a week, 150–250 minutes per week
> *or*
> STEPS PER DAY: approximately 10,000–13,999
> STRENGTH TRAINING: at least 2 times a week, a minimum of
> 6 exercises

Level 4 You're at Level 4 if you not only work out almost every day, but also cross-train (engage in multiple aerobic activities) to get added benefits and to lower your risk of an overuse injury. For example, three days a week you run, walk, or use the elliptical trainer at the gym, and on another two days, you do aerobic activities like swimming, riding a bike, or taking an aerobics class. Altogether you rack up about 250 minutes of aerobic exercise a week. You're also into strength-training and do so consistently three days a week, performing at least eight different exercises per session. On your easy day, you may take a yoga or stretch class.

AEROBIC EXERCISE: 5 times a week, at least 250–360 minutes per week

or

STEPS PER DAY: approximately 14,000–17,999

STRENGTH TRAINING: at least 3 times a week, a minimum of
8 exercises

Level 5 You're at Level 5 if exercise isn't just how you stay fit and healthy, it's a way of life. You may belong to a workout group, like a running, walking, or cycling club. Perhaps you challenge yourself by participating in races and competitions. You work out almost every day, maybe doing your main workout three times a week and cross-training three other days for a total of six hours of cardiovascular exercise a week. You've been strength-training for some time now, and you're up to at least ten different exercises, a minimum of three days a week.

AEROBIC EXERCISE: 6 times a week, 360 minutes or more per week

or

STEPS PER DAY: approximately 18,000 or above

STRENGTH TRAINING: at least 3 times a week, a minimum of
10 exercises

GOING TO THE NEXT LEVEL

Bumping up your activity level is a good idea no matter where you fall on the activity scale. But if you're at Level 0, it's critical. Your inactivity is a detriment to your health, and all the weight loss in the world isn't going to change that. If you fall into the completely inactive category, the thought of getting up and moving may never even cross your mind because you're so used to *not* moving. You will, though, have a better life if you consciously pursue activity. Don't be one of those people who wait five minutes in the car for someone to pull out of a parking space so that you'll only have to walk a few steps to your destination (you know who you are!).

I want to reiterate that physical activity is essential for long-term weight-loss success. There is nothing that offers as many benefits—from boosting the metabolism to preventing muscle loss—that directly affect your body weight and your well-being.

Going from activity Level 0 to Level 1 isn't difficult. Level 1 really doesn't even make any substantial demands on your schedule. Actually, it would be far better if you skipped Level 1 and just went straight to Level 2, which will give you far greater benefits than Level 1 and allow you to increase your calorie intake, too. Just be sure that if you've never engaged in formal workouts, or haven't done so in some time, you check with your physician before you jump to Level 2. If you were once an exerciser and stopped, you'll be surprised how easy it is to get back into it.

For those of you who are already exercising regularly and fall into Level 2 or above, your best bet is to move up one level at a time: increasing your exercise in increments will give your body time to adapt to the changes. But again, if you're at Level 0, it's okay to start engaging in formal workouts right away (after checking with your physician), and I encourage you to do just that.

I am going to add one caveat, no matter which activity level you choose: It's *very* important that you select a level of activity that you can see yourself doing for the rest of your life. Ideally, you'll exceed that level at some point, but what I don't want you to do is set your sights on a goal only to realize that it's impossible given your other time commitments and responsibilities. Just as the Best Life Diet shouldn't be something you go on, then go off of once you lose weight, activity should be something you work into your life permanently. If you're committed, there are plenty of ways to make room for exercise even if you have an extremely busy schedule. But if you're not willing to prioritize exercise right now, be honest with yourself. Choose to do as much as you're capable of doing instead of setting goals you can't meet.

It's not that I don't want you to aim high; on the contrary, I hope you will become an avid exerciser and perhaps even go all the way up to Level 5. But if you're unable to meet the activity goals that you set, you may end up doing no exercise at all, and that's the last thing you (or I) want to happen. Many people plan on going to the gym after work, get tied up, and skip it altogether. If they'd anticipated that they'd never leave the office early enough to make it to the gym, would feel too tired, would have to help their kids with homework, or any of the millions of other things that get in the way, then they could have taken a walk during lunchtime or before work and lifted a few weights in the morning before showering.

Don't let this happen to you. I like to exercise in the morning because there is less chance that something is going to prevent me from working out, as so often happens when you schedule exercise later in the day. You can even break up your workouts: do your cardio in the morning and strength-training later on if it makes it easier to get it all done. But if none of these scheduling ideas is going to make a difference for you, I'd rather have you set your sights lower and do *something*—even if it's a ten-minute walk around the neighborhood—rather than be overly ambitious and end up doing nothing at all. Get it right in the beginning so that you end up with an activity regimen that will last a lifetime.

Strategies for Increasing Your Activity

These are some basic guidelines for bumping up your activity level. To tap into a great array of strength-training exercises, cardio-workout ideas, and motivating tips, check out the complete exercise library at www .thebestlife.com. You'll also find research news about exercise and lots of advice on how to keep your workouts interesting.

As you read these strategies for increasing your activity, remember that you can gauge your aerobic exercise either in minutes per week or in steps per day or week. To move up to levels 3 to 5, you must include strength-training in your program in addition to your aerobic exercise/steps per day.

TO GO FROM LEVEL 0 TO LEVEL 1 . . .
You more than anyone else will benefit from having a pedometer, because the easiest and best way to move to Level 1 is simply to walk more. To gauge how much you're walking now and help you bump up that number, use the pedometer to measure how many steps you currently take in a day. For the first week, don't change your routine at all so that you can get a base-line number. Then gradually increase the number of steps you take. Your initial goal should be to get up to at least 3,500 steps and preferably 6,000 a day. Walk to the store for milk. Walk your kids to school. Walk down the hall to a colleague's office instead of communicating by using the phone or email. Walk around while you talk on the phone or give a presentation. Walk up stairs instead of using elevators and escalators (and if you're tak-

ing an escalator, walk up it; don't just stand there while it moves you). Walk to church or other community activities (and if it's too far to walk the whole way, park a good distance away and walk the remainder). As your pedometer will show you, you'll ultimately rack up some significant mileage, and that will translate into a significant number of calories burned.

Think, too, about how vigorously you move. One of the big differences between people who are overweight and people who aren't is that lean people not only fidget more, but also use more energy for everyday movements. For instance, someone who's energetic jumps up and picks up something that's fallen off her desk; someone who barely moves slides her chair over to grab it. The calorie-burning difference between the two ways of moving hardly seems like it would make one person skinny and another person heavier, but multiply it by the thousands of small moves you make each day, then by weeks, months, and years, and it all adds up to a big difference.

TO GO FROM LEVEL 1 TO LEVEL 2 . . .

You're about to make a substantial leap that may seem difficult at first. But don't worry. It's going to get easier, and you'll feel the rewards right away. You'll sleep better, feel better, and eventually even have more energy. (You may feel more tired than usual at first, but once the training effect kicks in and your body adapts, you'll definitely feel more lively.) Choose one or more types of aerobic exercise that you like—it could be walking, jogging, aerobic dance, spinning, salsa dancing, swimming, cycling, or kickboxing. Working out on machines like treadmills, stationary bikes, rowing machines, and elliptical trainers are a great way to go, too. Start by putting in as much time as you can comfortably handle—fifteen minutes a session, three sessions a week if you can do it, less if you can't. Each week add two minutes to your workouts until you reach thirty minutes per session; you'll then be meeting the ninety-minutes-a-week requirement in no time at all. Consider getting a workout partner, too: having someone to whom you're accountable can really help keep you on track. If you prefer to count steps to satisfy the aerobic requirement, increase your steps per day, working up to at least 6,000 daily.

TO GO FROM LEVEL 2 TO LEVEL 3 . . .

By adding strength-training to your regimen, you're doing both your muscles and your bones a big favor (strength-training is also one way to help prevent osteoporosis), and you're also moving up to a whole new level of commitment. Be creative about working strength-training into your schedule. Some people find that they prefer to complete their strength-training right after their aerobic workouts so that they can get everything out of the way in one fell swoop. Other people like to break their workouts up and do their aerobic/step component and strength-training on separate days, or on the same day but at separate times. One way isn't better than the other; whatever routine ensures that you're able to get everything done should be the one you choose.

To strength-train, start with one to two sets of six exercises (choose a selection that involves all the major muscle groups—see my website for some good options) at least two days a week. After six weeks, increase the number of sets you do to two or three. Also, gradually increase your aerobic sessions by two minutes per week, working toward a total of 150 minutes per week. If you're counting steps, increase your steps per day, working up to at least 10,000 to satisfy the aerobic requirement.

TO GO FROM LEVEL 3 TO LEVEL 4 . . .

At this stage, you should already be fairly fit, which will make advancing to the next level that much easier. Step up your strength-training regimen to include at least eight different exercises, two to three sets each, and do this a minimum of three days a week. Also, continue to boost your aerobic workout times by two minutes a week and raise the frequency of your workouts to six per week. Aim for a minimum total weekly aerobic exercise time of 250 minutes. This is a good time to diversify your workouts, too. Choose a second aerobic workout that you like and alternate between that and your original workout so that you're not overworking the same muscles. If you've been running on the treadmill, try the elliptical or rowing machines. If you've been cycling, why not try an aerobic dance or salsa class? If possible, also throw in a yoga, Pilates, or stretch class during the week. If you're counting steps, increase your steps per day, working up to at least 14,000 to satisfy the aerobic requirement.

TO GO FROM LEVEL 4 TO LEVEL 5 . . .

You're working out so often now that it's part of your lifestyle, and you're reaping significant benefits. But if you can do even more you'll be well rewarded. There's a body of new research indicating that people who do at least an hour of exercise a day make gains in everything from weight control to immunity.

One of the best ways to kick up your activity a degree is to test your skills. Enter 10Ks and half marathons, or maybe even full marathons. Join workout clubs; there are organizations for just about every possible activity, and these groups often train for both fun and serious competitions. To find a club, search the web or check with local sporting goods stores, which usually can point you in the right direction. To reach Level 5, you'll also be doing cardio exercise and raising your total aerobic workout time to six hours a week. If you're counting steps, increase your steps per day to at least 18,000 to satisfy the aerobic requirement. Increase your strength-training to a minimum of ten different exercises and the number of sets you do to three, at least three days a week. Now is also a good time to consider finding a training partner. You're putting a lot of hours into exercise, and having someone to talk to and encourage your effort will make the time go faster.

CHANGING THE WAY YOU EAT

Eat Three Meals plus at Least One Snack Daily

There's a good reason that every culture (at least every culture that I know of) goes by the three-meals-a-day rule. It's natural to get hungry every few hours, and although you may think you're doing yourself a favor by skipping a meal or even two, you're really only delaying your hunger, which can have very negative consequences. What's more, when your hunger catches up with you, it's likely to be intense, and it's hard to make good decisions about what to eat when your appetite is in overdrive. Ultimately, if you skip meals, you won't save calories; in fact, you'll most likely end up eating considerably more than you would if you'd eaten three meals a day.

So make eating three meals a priority and portion your meals out wisely. How should you divide them up? "Eat breakfast like a king, lunch like a prince, and dinner like a pauper" is the advice often given, and it has a lot of validity. Eating a big breakfast, a moderate lunch, and a small dinner is a great idea; the only problem is, for most people, it's not a realistic one. If you can ration your calories out that way, by all means go ahead, but I think what's more important is to make sure that you don't do the reverse: eat breakfast like a pauper (or not eat breakfast at all) and dinner like a king. In the evening, you're not likely to be very active, and your body (and your metabolism) is winding down, getting ready for sleep. Consuming most of your calories later in the day means that you're eating them when you're least able to burn them off. That alone could be a significant source of some of the extra pounds you're carrying. The bottom line is that you want to eat the bulk of your calories earlier in the day, which is the most efficient way to eat and the best way to ensure that you burn calories at an optimal level.

A happy medium between the "Eat breakfast like a king . . ." rule and what is probably feasible for you is to divide your calories fairly evenly among your meals. Plan to get 25 to 30 percent of your daily calories at each meal, with the remainder going toward your snack or snacks, which you'll see incorporated into the meal plans starting on page 161. This is not only a healthy way to distribute your calories and maximize calorie-burning, but it will also keep your insulin level from spiking, a process that signals your body to store fat. When you eat a large number of calories at one sitting, your body releases an unusually large amount of insulin. The insulin then shuttles blood sugar out of your bloodstream and deposits it as body fat: exactly what you *don't* want to happen.

Dividing up your calories wisely throughout the day will help you avoid the insulin response, keep your hunger at a reasonable level, and maximize your calorie-burning. There are, though, two aspects of your eating sched-ule that are particularly important, and because of that, I want to address each of them separately. The first is breakfast. The second is snacks.

EAT BREAKFAST!

I'm sure you've heard many times that breakfast is the most important meal of the day. This isn't just rhetoric someone invented to sell breakfast cereal. There are many good reasons—and some serious science—behind the rec-ommendation to start the day with a healthful meal. One of those reasons is that breakfast can have a significant impact on body weight. As someone who's trying to lose weight, you can't afford to dispense with breakfast.

Many people mistakenly believe that anytime you can refrain from eating, it's going to help you lose weight. But skipping meals doesn't contribute to weight loss in the long run, and this is particularly true when the meal you skip is breakfast. Perhaps you don't wake up hungry; *How nice,* you may think, *that I don't even have to try not to eat.* It sounds logical in theory, but you're not just missing out on calories. You're also missing out on a chance to rev up your metabolism and keep your appetite from raging out of control later in the day. Waking up without an appetite isn't "lucky" at all, and it's something you're going to have to work on changing. Having an eating cutoff time, which I'll go into on page 60, is going to help you wake up hungry, because you'll be going to bed already wanting a bite or two. If for some reason you still don't wake up with an appetite, give it an hour to develop, and if it doesn't, eat anyway. This is the only time I'm going to tell you to eat when you aren't at an appropriate hunger level (more of which you'll learn about in Phase Two). Breakfast is *that* important!

One of the things we know about the metabolism is that when you're asleep your calorie-burning rate slows way down. When you wake up in the morning, it starts to creep toward its normal speed, but the rise is very slow. Eating breakfast is like giving your metabolism a little jolt, causing it to rise faster and get to the business of burning calories at an optimal rate. A bowl of cereal, some toast, or a couple of eggs work to kick your metabolism into gear early in the day so that by the time the day is done, you'll have burned calories at a higher rate for more hours than if you'd waited until lunchtime to eat.

The jolt that breakfast gives to your metabolism is called the thermic effect of food. This refers to the increase in your metabolism that occurs whenever you eat. The thermic effect is not exclusive to breakfast; each time you eat, your metabolism increases slightly. That's the reason why eating three meals and a couple of snacks helps your metabolism stay revved up all day. But you particularly benefit from the thermic effect in the morning because it helps wake up your metabolism from its drowsy, post-sleep state.

Another reason that eating breakfast is essential to the weight-loss process is that it helps you tame your appetite throughout the rest of the day. If you forgo breakfast, chances are your appetite is going to roar to life right around the time you're perusing the lunch menu or gazing at the mac 'n' cheese peering out at you from behind the lunch counter. How

THE BEST LIFE BREAKFASTS

In Phase One, your main concern should be to make breakfast a habit. I want you to get used to eating soon after you wake up (or after activity if you're a morning exerciser) and avoid hitting the doughnut shop. Instead, consider one of the nine suggestions listed here (see the meal plans on pages 167–190 for more ideas). As you'll see, these meals are hardly spartan. In fact, they're as delicious as they are nutritious.

All of these breakfasts are rich in fiber, allowing you to get a big part of that daily requirement out of the way first thing in the morning. (The recommended amount of fiber is 25 g for women and 38 g for men, though most Americans consume only 15 g per day!) One thing you'll read repeatedly on these pages—because I really want to drive the point home— is that fiber helps you lose weight by making you feel fuller on fewer calories. Many high-fiber foods also help prevent spikes and dips in blood sugar, which helps keep your appetite under control.

And here's another great thing about these breakfast suggestions: each is calcium rich, providing at least 350 mg per serving.

NOTE: *How much of each breakfast selection you can have will depend on your activity level. See the breakfasts in the meal plan for your individual serving allowances.*

Cold Cereal Select a 100 percent whole grain cereal that's high in fiber (meaning it has at least 4 g of fiber per 100 calories) and low in sugar (preferably no more than 5 g). Or try one of my cereal combinations on pages 193–194. I love mixing cereals, which gives your bowl a variety of different tastes and textures and keeps it from becoming boring. Plus, different cereals bring different nutrients to the mix so it makes for a healthier bowlful. For most of you, 160–180 calories of cereal is a good portion. Douse your cereal with nonfat or 1 percent milk, or calcium-enriched soymilk; top it with fruit and, if you like, one to two tablespoons of heart-healthy nuts (walnuts, almonds, cashews, pecans, or peanuts).

Hot Cereal Here, too, choose a 100 percent whole grain variety like oatmeal. Start with one third to one half cup dry cereal and either cook it with nonfat or 1 percent milk or calcium-enriched soymilk instead of water, or add the milk to the cooked cereal. Top the cereal with fresh or dried fruit and, if you like, one to two tablespoons of nuts. I'm particularly a fan of McCann's Irish Oatmeal. Irish oatmeal has a rougher texture and takes longer to cook than regular oatmeal, but it's worth it!

Toast and Nut Butter Spread your 100 percent whole grain toast (or whole grain English muffin or bagel) with peanut butter, almond butter, cashew butter, or any other nut or soy butter. Add sliced apples or pears and a drizzle of honey, and wash it all down with a glass of nonfat or 1 percent milk or calcium-enriched soymilk. Check out the breakfasts on Day 3 and

Day 9 of the menu plan for portion guidance. If you haven't tried nut butters other than peanut butter before, then you may be turned off by their slightly runny consistency. But once you refrigerate them (which you'll need to do anyway to keep them fresh), they'll be thicker and closer to the texture of the peanut butter you're used to.

Eggs Serve one to two eggs with one slice of 100 percent whole grain toast or whole grain English muffin, fruit, and a glass of nonfat or 1 percent milk or calcium-enriched soymilk.

Bran or Whole Grain Muffins What could be easier than grabbing a muffin in the morning? Watch out, though, for those 800-calorie mega-muffins, and look instead for smaller, healthier muffins that weigh in at about 200 calories. Your best bet is probably to make them yourself. Try the Pumpkin Spice Muffins, page 196, or Pear Muffins, page 194. You can eat your muffins accompanied by a glass of nonfat or 1 percent milk or calcium-enriched soymilk and half a grapefruit.

NOTE: *Some Starbucks and similar cafés offer low-calorie bran muffins, but check the calorie counts online, since the muffins vary from café to café.*

Smoothie Smoothies never get boring because you can make them a hundred different ways. Blend together a small ripe banana, a cup of frozen berries or other fruit, a half cup of nonfat or 1 percent milk or calcium-enriched soymilk such as 8th Continent (which has an array of different flavors), a half cup of low-fat yogurt, a spoonful of honey, and wheat germ or ground flaxseed. (See pages 198–199, and 272 for some other smoothie recipes.)

Whole Grain Waffles and Pancakes Have whole grain waffles or pancakes that you make yourself from scratch or from a whole grain mix, and top them with yogurt, fruit, one to two tablespoons of heart-healthy nuts, and a drizzle of real maple syrup. The breakfast on Day 13 shows you appropriate portions for this breakfast.

Yogurt, Fruit, and Nuts Plain low-fat yogurt topped with fruit, nuts, a little honey, and, if you like, a spoonful of wheat germ or ground flaxseed (or a couple spoonfuls of low-fat granola) makes a terrific breakfast. And what could be easier? Look at breakfast on Day 4 for portion guidelines.

On-the-Go Breakfast When you don't even have time to sit down to a bowl of cereal, try this: stash a high-fiber bar (Fiber One chewy bars have a whopping 9 g of fiber) in your bag or briefcase; add a banana or an apple, a cup of nonfat or 1 percent milk or calcium-enriched soymilk (keep small cartons on hand or use a thermos), plus a small handful of nuts. Another alternative: one 11-ounce can of Slim-Fast Optima, any flavor; an apple; and one to two tablespoons of nuts.

vulnerable are you going to be to choosing the most fattening item you can find? Very. If you had eaten breakfast, however, you'd be less susceptible to temptation. In fact, studies show that people eat fewer calories throughout the day when they eat breakfast than when they don't. And British researchers recently found that not only did women consume fewer calories during the two weeks they ate breakfast, but they also had lower levels of LDL ("bad") cholesterol. One reason breakfast eaters may consume fewer calories overall may be that breakfast lends itself to high-fiber eating. Whole grain cereals, oatmeal, toast, waffles, and bran muffins as well as fruit are high in fiber and can be very filling, which can make you less likely to overeat later on in the day.

Most parents make it a point to get their kids to eat breakfast in the morning because they know that kids who go to class with something in their stomachs do better in school. Eating helps keep their minds sharp. As an adult, you should take advantage of that benefit, too—everyone can do with a little extra mental energy. Eating first thing is going to give you physical energy as well, and that's critical when you're trying to lose weight, because the more energy you have, the more you're going to move and the more calories you're going to burn. You'll have the stamina to make a hundred more calorie-burning moves a day, and over time that will translate into weight loss. So don't think of breakfast as just a meal that you can take or leave. Think of it as an integral part of your strategy to lose weight.

The Art of Snacking

If you've been on and off diets in the past, just the word *snack* may sound a little dangerous, suggesting that you're eating at a time when you shouldn't be. Certainly, if you snack all day long and your snacks are candy bars and fried tortilla chips, you're going to run into trouble. But when you snack moderately and intelligently, eating between meals will actually help you keep your food intake under control. I highly recommend that you have at least one snack per day, or two snacks if you feel you need them.

In the same way that breakfast can help you avoid becoming too hungry and, as a result, overindulging at subsequent meals, snacks help stabilize your blood sugar level and keep your appetite in check. A healthful

THE BEST LIFE SNACKS

The real overhaul of your meals and snacks will start when you enter Phase Two, but it won't hurt to start trying out these healthful 100–to–200-calorie snacks right now.

▶ 1 ounce whole grain pretzels with mustard

▶ 1 cup red pepper strips or celery sticks with $1/3$ cup of hummus

▶ $3/4$ cup carrots with 3 tablespoons of low-fat ranch dressing

▶ $3/4$ cup edamame

▶ 1 cup pineapple with 1–2 tablespoons of heart-healthy nuts

▶ 2–3 tablespoons of peanuts, almonds, walnuts, or cashews

▶ Trail mix: $1/4$ cup Multi-Bran Chex, 2 tablespoons of nuts, $1 1/2$ tablespoons of raisins or other dried fruit

CALCIUM-RICH SNACKS

▶ 1 cup Mocha Cooler (see recipe, page 271)

▶ Maple-Nut Yogurt: 1 teaspoon maple syrup and 1 tablespoon walnut pieces stirred into 6 ounces ($3/4$ cup) low-fat plain yogurt

▶ Milk and crackers: 60 calories' worth of high-fiber crackers (such as two pieces of Wasa Fiber Rye crispbread) spread with 2 teaspoons of jam, eaten with 1 cup nonfat or 1 percent milk or calcium-enriched soymilk

▶ Latte and nuts: 12-ounce skim milk latte and 8 almonds

▶ 1 ounce (1 slice) low-fat cheese on $1/2$ ounce whole grain crackers

▶ $3/4$ cup mixed berries with $3/4$ cup low-fat plain yogurt and 1 teaspoon of honey

▶ A fiber- and calcium-rich meal replacement, such as a Slim-Fast Optima shake, any flavor (11-ounce can)

snack will also help you stay energized and provide your metabolism with a little boost (the thermic effect at work again). The key, of course, is to snack wisely, which is why I've provided some wholesome snack suggestions here, plus more in the menu plans starting on page 161. Among the recommendations are a number of calcium-rich snacks. If you incorporate one of these snacks into your diet per day and also have one of my calcium-rich breakfast suggestions, are taking one of my suggested multivitamin and mineral supplements, and are eating a balanced diet, you'll meet your calcium requirement and won't need to worry about it the rest of the day. (If, however, you're over fifty, you may still need a supplement; see page 67.)

Like the rest of your diet, the recommended number of calories you "spend" on snacks will depend on your activity level. If, for instance, you're a woman at Activity Level 0, you'll have less calories per day to devote to snacks than a woman at Activity Level 3 (look through the menu plans and you'll see the differences). Check the list on page 59 for great snack ideas.

Stop Eating at Least Two Hours Before Bedtime

If you're familiar with any of my other books, you'll know that I'm a stickler for this rule: **STOP EATING AT LEAST TWO HOURS BEFORE YOU GO TO BED.** This is part of a strategy to get you to shift your calorie consumption toward the earlier part of the day, as well as one of the most effective and easiest eating habits you can establish. Some people don't understand why I'm so wedded to it, and they often ask, "If a calorie is a calorie, what does it matter what time of day you eat it?" Here's what I tell them: It's true that whether you eat, say, a cup of low-fat lemon yogurt at 11 A.M. or 11 P.M., it's still going to have about 200 calories. But when you eat that yogurt in the morning, your metabolism speeds up a bit, maximizing the rate at which your body burns calories. At night, though, your body has already shifted into low gear in preparation for sleep, so you're not going to get much of a metabolic boost from late-night eating.

You'll find that I keep returning to these little variations in calorie use again and again. That's because they really do make a difference. Nobody gains a lot of weight overnight; it happens over time. If you were eating huge ice-cream sundaes every night, you probably wouldn't be surprised if you gained weight. But if you don't really understand why you've put on excess pounds over the years, it may be because the habits and actions that got you there—taking the elevator instead of the stairs and/or the extra sour cream on your nachos—seemed so inconsequential. What I'm trying to do is draw your attention to all of the seemingly minor, but ultimately significant, factors that affect your body weight. The good news is that you can do something about all of them, and this one in particular—eating no later than two hours before bedtime—can have a real impact on your weight. Many of my clients have found that just having an eating cutoff time alone has helped them reach their weight-loss goals.

There are a few other reasons why it's important to have a cutoff time. For one thing, it's not healthy to go to bed on a full stomach. Digestion essentially shuts down when you're sleeping, and it's in your body's best interest to speed food through the digestive tract so that you have as little contact with waste as possible.

The main reason that we eat (though obviously not the only one) is to fuel our bodies. Food gives us energy. When you eat earlier in the day (especially when you eat a well-balanced combination of nutritious foods), the food you consume peps you up so that you *do* take the stairs, you *do* run for the bus, you *do* walk to the video store instead of hopping in the car. Maybe you even go to the gym. But when you eat in the evening close to the time you're going to call it a day, your body is already winding down and getting ready for sleep. The body at rest doesn't need much fuel. Consequently, that energy doesn't get used and is stored in the body as fat.

I believe that there's also a psychological side to this. When you eat earlier in the day, you're more conscious about burning it off. It goes through your head (*Hmm, I had a pretty big sandwich for lunch*) and inspires you to do something about it (*Better go for a walk after work*). But after 9 P.M., frankly, who has the energy to care? I highly doubt you're going to race off to the twenty-four-hour gym as penance for a late-night sandwich. So, you see, even if calories don't change in the evening, *human beings* change. It's in our nature to want to shut down after a certain hour. That puts you in danger of putting on pounds and certainly makes it harder to lose them.

If you feel a little tug of hunger, as though maybe you could eat a little something before you go to bed, that's a sign that you've let enough time lapse after your last meal or snack. When your body tells you that it wants food, it's saying, in essence, "Feed me, or I'll go into your fat stores and feed myself." Great! That's what you want to happen. So if you go to bed wanting a little something, you're right on target. And if you go to bed slightly hungry, you're going to wake up hungry and want breakfast. And that, as you now know, is going to help you stick to the three-meals-a-day rule.

There are going to be evenings when you're going to feel that tug of hunger powerfully and find it hard to ignore. If it's true hunger because you haven't eaten all day, then a 6-ounce yogurt, a banana, or a slice of whole wheat toast thinly spread with peanut butter should satisfy you. The next day, make sure to eat three meals and a snack so you're not hungry at night. If it's ice cream or other comfort foods you're craving, then this is the time to fix yourself a cup of soothing herbal tea like chamomile or peppermint or green tea (one of my current favorites is Lipton Pyramid Green Tea with Mandarin Orange Flavor). Pull out your journal and use this time to write about your life. Refer back to the questions beginning on page 26 or go to my website for some emotional eating/self-discovery exercises. This is a golden opportunity for you to think about what has pulled you toward food in the past and what needs to happen in your life to make food less of a draw. Ask yourself what else you could do instead of eating that would benefit your life. Replace the restless energy that usually leads you to the refrigerator with time spent improving your life.

Stay Hydrated

For a while, drinking water was all the rage. You couldn't go anywhere without seeing people dragging along a bottle of spring water. Suddenly, vending machines that sold only soda offered water, too. Then came the backlash and inevitable controversy. Some people began wondering whether we really needed to drink so much water. I, for one, think we do. Everybody should drink at least six 8-ounce glasses (48 ounces) of water a day, and it's particularly important if you're trying to slim down.

For one thing, all physiological processes—including digestion and burning calories—work better when the body is adequately hydrated. Ironically, a lot of diets, especially low-carb, high-protein diets, are geared toward making you lose water. That's why they offer such rapid results (that's also one of the reasons why when you go off them, you gain weight so quickly—the water simply comes back). But it's not water you want to get rid of; it's fat, and from a fat-loss standpoint, dehydrating yourself really works against you. If you're dehydrated, you're not going to burn calories at an optimal level, and that's going to make it hard to lose body fat.

Some recent research from the University of North Carolina–Chapel

Hill also suggests that people who drink an average of 6½ cups of water during the day consume close to 200 fewer calories per day. The water drinkers in the study tended to have healthier eating habits and drank less soda. It's impossible to say if it was the water itself that quenched their appetite and made them less likely to eat, but I do think it shows that drinking adequate amounts of water goes hand in hand with healthful eating.

If you're following a diet that's high in fruits and vegetables (and if you're not now, you will be by Phase Three), that's also going to help you stay hydrated, but I still recommend getting at least six glasses of noncarbonated water a day. And that's especially true if you consume a lot of caffeine, because caffeine causes water loss. There's no reason to go overboard—if six cups of water is good, twelve cups isn't necessarily better (unless it's a very hot day and you've been exercising hard)—but it's smart to get at least the minimum for both physiological and practical reasons. Consider, for instance, that drinking water is distracting. If you've got a water bottle in your hand, you're going to feel less inclined to dip your fingers into a bag of chips. And while water isn't as filling as food, it still dampens the appetite for a little while, and that can help you forgo some of the calories you may have otherwise consumed.

There are times you may feel as though your body is craving food when in fact it's craving water; that's one of the dangers of being dehydrated. Dehydration also makes exercising harder. When you work out, your muscles actually hold on to water (see page 18 for an explanation), a sign that they need to be hydrated to meet the demands you're placing on them. When you short them of water, you're preventing them from operating at full capacity and upping the likelihood that you'll fatigue faster as you exercise. What's more, your body needs extra water to cool itself off through perspiration while you're working out.

Keep in mind that iced tea, juice, and other beverages shouldn't take the place of your 48 ounces of water. No matter what else you drink, have your water, too. Get used to having a glass at every meal. If it's really hard for you to drink so much unflavored liquid, try herbal iced tea, carbonated waters, or some of the flavor-infused waters on the market now (see page 167 for some suggestions). Just a squirt of lemon, lime, grapefruit, or even a little tangerine juice can help plain water go down a little easier, too.

Eliminate Alcohol, for Now

A healthful diet can include alcohol, and yours certainly can—once you get into Phase Three. For now, though, avoid all alcohol. One reason alcohol and weight loss don't mix is because alcohol adds extra calories to your diet—it weighs in at 7 calories per gram, while carbohydrates and protein only weigh in at 4 calories per gram (fat has 9 calories per gram). A five-ounce glass of wine has 100 calories, a twelve-ounce glass of beer has 148 calories, and that small 4½-ounce piña colada has 262 calories. Alcohol is also absorbed quickly into your bloodstream, and as a depressant, it slows down everything in your body, including your metabolism. Plus, if you've had a few, will you be able to make good decisions about what you eat? From my vantage point, the inebriation factor, even if it's slight, keeps many people from sticking to a well-balanced diet.

I've also found that many people are simply not aware of how much they're drinking, and it takes abstaining for a while to get them attuned to their intake. If you don't drink much, eliminating alcohol probably won't be much of a problem for you, but if you're fond of a nightly drink (or more), this is a good chance to reassess your approach to alcohol.

There's been a big push lately to include alcohol, especially wine, in one's diet because of its potential to lower the risk of heart disease. This benefit may eventually prove to be a powerful one (we still don't know for sure); however, if you don't consume wine, then you aren't necessarily going to be missing out on a good way to protect your heart: exercise does the same thing. And we *know* that exercise benefits and protects the heart. What's more, if alcohol makes you tired and groggy and keeps you from taking your morning walks or making it to the gym, it is going to do more harm to your heart than good. Plus, one of the best things you can do for your heart if you're overweight is to shed pounds. If alcohol interferes with that goal, then it's not offering you much protection.

So take a time-out from alcohol for now. In Phase Three, you can reassess how much it means to you and work it back into your diet using your Anything Goes calories.

Bolster Your Diet with Daily Supplements

Nutrition is still a relatively new science, but researchers are making some incredible advances. One day your doctor will probably be able to look at your DNA and give you a tailor-made prescription for the exact quantities of the exact nutrients you need for optimal health. Right now, however, nobody really knows the precise needs of each individual, so the best you can do is try to cover all your bases with a multivitamin and mineral supplement. This is particularly important when you're cutting calories, because when you eat less, you also reduce the amount of vitamins and minerals you take in. Supplements aren't a replacement for healthful food, but we don't always get as many nutrients from food as we'd like. Many fruits and vegetables are shipped cross-country. If you combine the time it takes for them to get to stores with the time they sit on store shelves, there is a lot of opportunity for certain nutrients in these healthy foods to degrade. Modern processing and farming techniques have reduced the nutritional quality that used to be inherent in many foods. If you remember what your average supermarket tomato tasted like when you were a kid and what it tastes like today, you know what I'm talking about, because flat flavor is often a sign of fewer nutrients.

Taking a multivitamin and mineral supplement is like a nutritional insurance policy, and it may even lower your risk of disease. I'm going to also recommend that you take an omega-3 fatty acid supplement and, if necessary, a calcium supplement, too.

If you smoke (which I hope you don't, or won't for much longer) or are on birth control pills, taking extra vitamin C is a good idea. Some people find that it helps them get over colds more quickly, too. In any case, an extra 500 mg per day can't hurt.

CHOOSING A DAILY MULTIVITAMIN

Look for a multivitamin that has close to 100 percent of the daily value for most of the "big" nutrients: vitamins A, C, E, D, and folic acid, along with the minerals iron, zinc, copper, and manganese. A good supplement will also have vitamin K, selenium, magnesium, chromium, and some calcium (about 150 mg). Pass on those supplements that have lots of extraneous additives like green tea, borage, amino acids, and digestive enzymes. They

NOTE: I can vouch for the examples of good brand-name multis as of the publication date of this book, but check the labels carefully, as products may change.

just leave less room in the pills for the nutrients you really need. Also, skip supplements with more than 18 mg iron, 23 mg zinc, or more than 10,000 IU of vitamin A or 15,000 IU of beta-carotene; in these cases, more is not a good thing. One last piece of advice: try to find a supplement that you take once a day. If you forget to take a vitamin that requires multiple doses, you won't get the full benefit, and a multiple-dose vitamin may cost more money.

Women and men have slightly different nutritional requirements, and these requirements change a little as you get older, so check the label of your vitamins to make sure you're getting what you need.

WOMEN Age fifty or under: Have 18 mg iron, at least 12 mcg vitamin K, and at least 400 mcg folic acid. Examples: One-A-Day Women's, Rite Aid Whole Source, or Theragran-M Premier.

MEN Age fifty or under: Have no more than 10 mg iron and at least 12 mcg vitamin K. Examples: One-A-Day Men's Health Formula, Theragran-M Advanced Formula, or Kroger Thera Plus.

WOMEN AND MEN Over age fifty: Have no more than 10 mg iron, at least 12 mcg vitamin B12, and 10 mcg vitamin K. Examples: Nature Made for Her 50+, Nature Made for Him 50+, or One-A-Day 50 Plus.

OMEGA-3 FATTY ACIDS

This is the first time I've put omega-3 fatty acids on my recommended supplements list. While I used to eat fish several times a week to get my omega-3s (they're particularly prevalent in fatty fish like salmon, herring, mackerel, sardines, and, to a lesser extent, tuna), I find that I'm eating less fish these days because of concerns about pollution, heavy metals, and overfishing. So now I rely more on a supplement to get my omega-3s. It's pretty clear that omega-3s reduce blood clotting, lowering the risk of heart attack and stroke. They also lower blood triglycerides and decrease inflammation, both of which can contribute to heart disease. Interestingly, some research suggests that omega-3s may improve mood, too. One British study even found that two-thirds of depressed patients who took omega-3 supplements had a 50 percent reduction in feelings of sadness and pessimism. That's as good a reason as any to try them out. (Note that if you're on warfarin or another blood-thinner, check with your doctor before taking any omega-3 supplement. One way they help reduce heart disease risk is by thinning the blood, which helps prevent clots. But if you're already on medication to do this, then the omega-3 supplement could cause excessive bleeding.)

The two most potent types of omega-3s are those found in fish oil: eicosapentaenoic acid (EPA) and docosahexaenoic acid (DHA). Alpha-linoleic acid (ALA), found in vegetarian sources of omega-3s, such as flaxseed, is also beneficial, but not as effective as EPA and DHA. If you choose to take an omega-3 supplement, your daily dose should be 1 g a day, divided roughly equally between EPA and DHA. Check the supplement label carefully; often it takes two or three tablets to get the full dose. If you have high blood triglycerides, ask your doctor about taking two to four grams of omega-3s daily, as suggested by the American Heart Association. Look for supplements that have been distilled to ensure that they're free of mercury and other pollutants. You can also get more omega-3s in your diet by eating eggs from chickens fed omega-3-rich feed, walnuts, flaxseed, soy and canola oils, and omega-3-enriched products like Barilla PLUS pasta.

CALCIUM

One of the best things you can do to prevent bone loss as you age is to strength-train. Another is to include adequate amounts of calcium in your diet, especially if you have a family history of osteoporosis. If you eat one of the calcium-rich Best Life breakfast recommendations (listed on pages 56–57) and at least one calcium-rich snack, eat a nutritious diet, and take a multi that contains calcium, you don't have to worry about taking a calcium supplement if you're under the age of fifty. You'll get close to the 1,000 mg of calcium you need to meet the recommended daily requirement (you can also get calcium from other nondairy sources like broccoli, kale, Swiss chard, almonds, and fortified foods like orange juice). If you're over the age of fifty, I recommend that you take 500 mg of some form of calcium daily. Because calcium absorption falls as you get older, and for women bone loss speeds up after menopause, the recommended amount of calcium climbs from 1,000 mg to 1,200 mg a day.

There are many different types of calcium supplements, including calcium carbonate, calcium citrate, and calcium lactate. Despite claims to the contrary, there's not much difference in how well the body absorbs the different types of calcium, especially if you take the supplement with a meal, which will help increase absorption. Get a chewable tablet or one that dissolves in water to ensure that it breaks down. I personally prefer calcium carbonate (such as Tums) or calcium citrate (such as Citracal).

Judging Your Success

After four weeks in Phase One, ask yourself the following questions:

▶ Did you successfully increase your activity?

▶ Have you managed to consistently eat three meals a day and one or two snacks?

▶ Have you stuck to an eating cutoff time?

▶ Do you wake up hungry for breakfast?

▶ Have you been drinking lots of water but no alcohol?

▶ Are you taking a daily multivitamin/mineral supplement?

▶ Finally, what do you weigh now?

If you're able to answer the first six questions with a yes, then it's a good sign that you're easing into new lifestyle habits and that you're ready to move on to Phase Two. But use your weight as the final criterion. If you lost about a pound or more a week, you should consider staying in Phase One for two or three more weeks. Just making some lifestyle changes alone has helped you cut enough calories to put you into an energy deficit, and that's great news. Don't be disappointed if you were all ready to move on to Phase Two; you're doing really well. One change you should make if you decide to keep going in Phase One is to monitor your weight once a week. Once you stop losing weight, you'll know it's time for you to move on.

If you weigh yourself after the first four weeks and the scale indicates that you didn't lose much weight, I don't want you to be discouraged. The point of Phase One is to make an investment in yourself that is going to pay off later. You've been preparing your body for the aggressive weight loss that's to come in the next stage of this program.

So, if you made all the lifestyle changes and are holding steady at about the same weight, move on to Phase Two. If you weren't able to make all the lifestyle changes—regardless of whether the numbers on the scale dropped or not—consider staying in Phase One until you get comfortable with all of these new habits.

PHASE TWO

▶ The investments you made in yourself in Phase One—especially moving more and restructuring how you eat—will have both immediate and lasting benefits. While in Phase One, you began losing some body fat and, most important, your body was being primed for the significant and consistent weight loss to come. By the time you reach Phase Two, you'll have built a great racecar; now you're going to take it out for a drive.

There are several changes you're going to make during this phase that will get the pounds to drop off more aggressively now than at any other time during this program. You're going to change what you eat, though in ways that I don't think you'll find overly demanding. I'm going to ask you to eliminate just six foods from your diet: soda, foods that contain trans fats, fried foods, white bread, and high-fat milk and yogurt. You're also going to begin practicing portion control. If you're like most people, that's probably going to be your biggest challenge; however, this phase is also devoted to introducing you to effective ways to monitor and control your appetite. When you don't feel hungry all the time and are more in touch with how hungry you actually are, portion control is going to come naturally.

Understanding and controlling your hunger is a major part of this phase because this too often goes unaddressed. Nothing can doom a diet faster than a strong desire to eat! Hunger is, after all, one of the most basic of human urges. In many diet programs, hunger is rarely ever mentioned, as if it will go away by itself. But feelings of hunger are something all of us have to live with to some extent (especially when reducing calories), and it's important to acknowledge that those feelings can be a major obstacle to weight loss. At the same time, food cravings and the desire to eat more than necessary is not an insurmountable problem. While the mechanisms involved in appetite are complex, you actually have more control over your hunger than you may think.

Following the guidelines in Phase One should have helped you regulate your appetite to some degree so that by the time you get to Phase Two, you may already be struggling less with hunger. One of the benefits of eating regular meals and snacks is that you address your hunger before you get to the point of feeling famished and overeating. Establishing an eating cutoff time also improves hunger control because it ensures that you wake up wanting breakfast; as noted in Phase One, eating breakfast helps normalize your appetite throughout the rest of the day.

In Phase Two, you will continue the process of learning to control your hunger. As you gain greater understanding of why you may have an oversized appetite—and whether that appetite is truly a reflection of your physical hunger, your emotions, and your routine, or simply the cues you get from the abundance of food around you—you're going to find that

PHASE TWO

TIME FRAME: A minimum of four weeks

WEIGH IN: The first day of this phase, then again once a week

FOCUS: Significant and consistent weight loss brought about by understanding and controlling your hunger and making a few dietary changes

OBJECTIVES:

▶ Build on the changes you made in Phase One:

  ▷ Live an active life

  ▷ Stop eating at least two hours before bedtime

  ▷ Eat three meals, including a nutritious breakfast, plus at least one snack daily

  ▷ Stay hydrated

  ▷ Bolster your diet with daily supplements

▶ Increase your activity at least one level (optional)

▶ Understand the physical nature of your hunger

▶ Understand the emotional reasons for your hunger

▶ Use the hunger scale

▶ Eat reasonable portions

▶ Remove six empty or problem foods from your diet

JUDGING YOUR SUCCESS: Check in at week four to see whether you're ready to move on there are several tactics you can use to diminish your desire to eat too much and/or too often. The information in this section is also geared toward helping you discover foods that fill up your stomach at a low-calorie cost. These foods are relatively low in calories themselves, *plus* they dampen your appetite for extended periods of time so that you ultimately eat fewer calories throughout the day.

The two other main objectives in this phase are to practice portion control and to take six foods out of your diet that add too many empty calories or put your health at risk—or, in many cases, both. When you eliminate these foods and replace them with less fattening and more nutritious alternatives, your weight loss will accelerate. If you've already taken these foods out of your diet or if they never really figured into what you eat on most days, portion control is going to be the biggest factor spurring on your weight loss. Either way, and especially if you'll be making both changes, you should see the pounds begin to drop off at the reasonable rate of 1 to 2 pounds a week.

During this phase, you'll also begin transitioning your taste buds for the changes that follow in Phase Three. You're moving toward adopting the healthy diet you're going to have for life. Letting your sense of taste evolve over time is a far more effective approach to healthful eating than waking up one day and shocking your palate with a completely new diet. Going cold turkey to stop smoking may be a good idea, but it's a strategy that doesn't translate so well when it comes to diet. Besides, quitting smoking involves giving up one thing—tobacco—while eating involves making many changes. Plus, food needs to be in your life while smoking definitely does not. While you're learning to live with changes in some areas of your diet, it's still possible take comfort in those foods that remain familiar to you until you begin replacing them in Phase Three.

I think it's important to be realistic about transforming your diet. Most Americans' taste buds have been bombarded with intense flavors because most foods these days, whether you buy them from supermarkets or from restaurants, are saturated with the tastes humans are predisposed to prefer: sweetness (which we get in the form of both regular sugar and sugar substitutes), saltiness, and fattiness. The Best Life Diet is designed to reduce the amounts of sweet, salty, and fatty foods you consume over time, but I also want to acknowledge that it's not easy to give up those flavors.

Most people go through at least a little withdrawal. It is, however, possible to wean yourself down to a healthier intake of these foods, and that should be your ultimate goal.

In a perfect world, all of us would have perfect diets. In the real world, most of us continue refining our diets on an ongoing basis. I'm still working on tweaking my own diet in lots of different ways, including getting even more of the sugar out and getting more whole grains in. Again, it's a process, but consider the changes you'll be making in this phase as a big step forward.

TIME FRAME

Like Phase One, Phase Two is a minimum of four weeks long. And as with Phase One, you may want to stay in this phase until you're either at your goal weight or at least within 20 pounds of it. There's a section at the end of this chapter that will point you in the right direction as to when it's time to transition into Phase Three.

I don't want you to get locked into a time frame if it turns out that you either haven't been able to incorporate all of the Phase Two guidelines into your life or that you are doing so well with them that it's best to sit tight and take advantage of your success. Wait until you make your success assessment at the end of four weeks to decide whether or not you're ready to move on.

WEIGH IN

In this phase, you'll weigh yourself once a week; however, I still want you to be wary of tying your emotions to the scale. Keep in mind that even when water-weight fluctuations become less severe, weight loss hardly ever occurs in a completely straight line. Don't be too hard on yourself if the numbers on the scale don't live up to your expectations week after week. Use your weigh-in results as an opportunity to look over the changes you've made and see where you may need to fine-tune your efforts.

When weighing yourself, remember to

1 use the same scale,

2 weigh yourself at approximately the same time and on the same day of the week, and

3 wear the same amount of clothing.

PHASE TWO OBJECTIVES

Build on the Changes You Made in Phase One

By now you should be in the habit of eating three meals and at least one snack a day, drinking at least six glasses of water, and taking your vitamin supplement daily. Your eating cutoff time should be in place and alcohol, for the time being, is off your roster of permissible beverages. Except for drinking alcohol, which you have the choice to add back into your diet in Phase Three (using your Anything Goes calories), the changes you made in Phase One are changes that should be part of your permanent Best Life routine. Don't get the idea that the modifications you're going to adopt in Phase Two supplant those from Phase One. The guidelines from Phase One are part of the foundation of this program and are the rules you should follow even if, for some reason, you falter for a time. Phase One is what's going to keep you grounded and, if ever necessary, help you get back on track.

Increase Your Activity at Least One Level (Optional)

While this objective is optional, I do strongly suggest that you try and increase your activity level again. My strongest recommendation is that you move as much as possible and live an active life; by Phase Two, you should be at least at Activity Level 1 and preferably at Level 2. But for all the reasons I gave in Phase One—the more you're moving your body, the better it will be for your health, the more food you'll be able to eat and the easier the weight-loss process will be—I want to encourage you to kick it up another notch.

Because you increased your activity in Phase One, moving to the next tier will be less difficult; your body has already adapted to some of the demands of exercise. And remember, you will be rewarded nicely for your efforts. The activity will give your metabolism another boost, further increasing the number of calories you burn throughout the day and helping to advance your weight loss during this phase (while still allowing you to eat a little bit more). As you'll also learn in the upcoming sections, exercise can help you curb your appetite, too. So see how much more activity you can reasonably accommodate in your life and adjust accordingly.

APPETITE CONTROL

Understand the Physical Nature of Your Hunger

Eating is meant to be one of life's great pleasures, but the pleasure you get from eating is also a survival tool, meant to ensure that you'll want to eat and therefore stay alive. Pleasure, though, is just one of several different physiological mechanisms devoted to making you desire food. And not only do those mechanisms make you want to eat, but they also make you want to eat the foods that will sustain you the longest: those with a lot of calories.

The reasons for why you get hungry and what makes you feel full are complicated. Scientists are just now beginning to get a handle on the intricacies of appetite, and their work is far from done. In recent years, though, they've been able to tell us quite a bit about what causes hunger to strike and how the body turns the appetite on as well as off.

Most of the time your thoughts turn to food because your brain is getting a variety of different signals from your body urging you to eat. One of these signals comes from a hormone called ghrelin, which is produced when your stomach empties. When you begin eating, your brain gets the message to keep going. It's almost as if there were a going-out-of-business sale on your plate, with your body saying, "There's food here! Get it while you can!" Gradually, some of the mechanisms that turn off your appetite start to chime in. As your stomach fills with food, the expansion triggers the nerves in your stomach's walls to send signals telling your brain to slow down. At the same time, ghrelin production ends, and that, along with the release of other hormones, sends the same message, letting your brain know you can stop eating now. Further input is received by a hormone called leptin, which originates within your fat cells. Leptin clues your brain into how much body fat you're carrying; if the level is high enough, it contributes to the symphony of messages telling you that you can leave the dinner table.

It's really a very elegant and efficient system, except that there are all kinds of things that can conspire to throw it off. One problem is that it can take as long as twenty minutes for the I'm-full message to reach your brain, which potentially means (and usually does) that you'll keep eating beyond the point that you need to. Fortunately, that's a problem that you can override by pausing before you have a second helping or continue with dessert. Stopping to let your brain catch up with your body is one of the most powerful tools you have for dealing with physical hunger, and I'll talk more about that later in this chapter.

The other glitches aren't as easy to correct. Some research, for instance, has shown that many obese people are resistant to leptin; their brains don't get the message that they have enough body fat, which may be one reason they have trouble controlling their appetite. Also, whenever you lose weight, your body will try to get back to its set point—the weight range that you're programmed to maintain—by changing levels of some of the hormones that control your appetite. Leptin production will drop so that your brain doesn't get the don't-eat signal it normally would, while ghrelin production will rise so that it gets more of the do-eat message. If you've ever found that after losing a certain amount of weight you suddenly feel like eating everything in sight, this could be one of the reasons.

Complicating matters is the fact that hunger and food cravings are also triggered by the motivation and reward centers of your brain. Instead of inducing you to eat because your stomach is empty, certain brain chemicals encourage you to eat for pure pleasure. "Go out, get something delicious and devour it," they say. "It's going to feel really good!"

And, of course, it does, but this isn't just hedonism. Like our ancestors who lived through times when food could be scarce, we're hardwired to desire foods high in calories, even though we don't need to pack in as many calories as possible every chance we get for survival purposes. Even so, the motivation and reward centers of the brain still operate on the assumption that the more calories, the better, which likely explains why foods like cookies, ice cream, and chips are so alluring.

Some people, of course, have a harder time resisting high-calorie foods than others, and now scientists are discovering that there may be a physiological reason why. One of the most interesting recent findings is that the brain chemistry of some obese people is similar to the brain chemistry of drug addicts and alcoholics. Both groups of people have lower levels of receptors for dopamine, a chemical that is part of the brain's motivation-and-reward system. Dopamine drives you to grab for something that will bring you pleasure. If you're low on receptors for the chemical, it may be that you don't process pleasurable stimuli, whether from food, alcohol, or drugs, as easily as the average person, so it takes more of them to bring you to the point where your brain says "I've had enough" and signals your body to put on the brakes. Another possible explanation is that if you're short on dopamine receptors, then you won't be as receptive to other pleasures in life, making you vulnerable to the things that *do* give you pleasure—in this case, food.

For a long time, people who said they were addicted to food were dismissed as overstating the case, but this new research lends some credibility to the argument that certain people have physiological differences that make them more susceptible to overeating. Another possible difference between food addicts and regular eaters is their levels of serotonin, a brain chemical that also affects appetite. Serotonin affects mood, and many antidepressants work by readjusting the level of serotonin in the brain. It's also believed to activate brain chemicals that depress appetite and block those that increase appetite. Some researchers believe that serotonin, or, more specifically, lack of serotonin, is behind cravings for cookies, candy, bread, and other sugary and/or starchy foods. These foods boost the release of serotonin, increasing the sense of well-being. The serotonin theory, though, is complex, because drugs that increase serotonin levels such as antidepressants tend to promote weight *gain,* not loss.

Scientists are also looking at the connection between stress and comfort foods. So far, studies seem to indicate that foods full of fat and sugar actually put the brakes on the release of stress hormones. But you probably don't need a study to tell you that. If you hit your kitchen cupboards the minute you get home after a stressful day, you know all too well that comfort foods do just that—comfort us.

Controlling Physical Hunger

Understanding the inner workings of your appetite can be a lot of information to process, but I hope that comprehending what's going on in your body will help you gain greater insight into the weight-loss process. Your body has a system for minimizing weight loss (believe it or not, it also has a system for minimizing gain, too), but by adopting the changes set out for you in this program, you will be able to override some aspects of that system and lose the weight you need to.

Exercise, for instance, activates some of the same pleasure circuitry in the brain as food. By producing pleasure-inducing brain chemicals called endorphins, activity can provide some of the comfort you may otherwise get from eating. Research also suggests that exercise can increase the number of dopamine receptors you have, good news if you have a naturally low count. (Short of going to a lab for expensive tests, there's no way to know whether you do or not; however, if many people in your family struggle with overeating and obesity or addiction, it may be a sign that you do have fewer dopamine receptors than normal.) These are just a few other reasons why it's to your advantage to try and increase your activity level as much as you possibly can.

By cleaning up your diet, as you'll do gradually on this program, you're also going to be taking an important step toward controlling your hunger. One of the theories about why people eat too much junk food is that when you consume an abundance of fat and sugar, it disrupts all the signals that carry out normal appetite regulation. By reducing the amount of fatty and sugary foods in your diet, you're going to bring your body's hunger and satiety network back into balance.

The healthful foods that replace the junk food in your diet are also going to bring their own appetite-control benefits to the table. Many of these foods will be high in fiber and/or water. Fiber, a type of carbohydrate that helps give certain foods their bulk and that can't be digested by the body, helps you stay fuller longer. Fiber slows down digestion so that your blood sugar level stays elevated and delays the release of some of the hormones that signal your brain that it's time to eat again. As an added bonus, foods rich in fiber tend to be lower in energy density: the fiber takes up space, but adds no calories.

Your diet should contain at least 25 g of fiber daily if you're a woman, 38 g if you're a man. All the breakfasts in the Best Life Diet Meal Plans (pages 167–190) have 9 or more grams of fiber; all the lunches and dinners contain 8 or more grams. I've also given you some high-fiber snack options on my list of snacks (page 59).

Water-rich foods also help you feel full on fewer calories, according to extensive research at Pennsylvania State University. Water, like fiber, adds bulk to food and lowers the foods' calorie counts, which is why vegetables and fruit—the foods highest in water—tend to be less energy dense than other foods. The Best Life Diet urges you to eat lots of salads and soups, two dishes that are particularly water-rich and have been shown to help people lower their calorie intake when they're eaten as an appetizer. If you start a meal with soup, choose one that has 100 calories or less per cup. Progresso, for instance, has about thirty-two soups that fit the bill.

Because most high-fiber and water-rich foods are fairly low in calories, they also allow you to eat more than foods that are energy dense (fatty foods like nuts, for instance, are considered energy dense because there are a lot of calories packed into each individual nut). This can help you deal with hunger, too, because hunger and satisfaction are often tied to expectations. If you're used to eating a large bowl of food but are served a small one, you may still feel hungry after you've finished eating its contents, even if what's in the small bowl has more calories. Being able to eat bigger portions should help you feel less deprived while still allowing you to cut calories.

There is, of course, a limit to how big your portions should be, and I don't want to give you the idea that portion sizes don't matter, even if you're eating relatively low-calorie foods. One of the biggest contributors to the obesity crisis sweeping this country is that many people consume portions that are simply too large. It's an important issue, and I address it at length on pages 95–98. I do, however, want to acknowledge that we now live in a world where restaurants think nothing of offering (and many people think nothing of consuming) 42-ounce sodas and steaks the size of hardcover books. It's easy to become accustomed to big portions; after a time, your brain associates them with satisfaction and anything less seems skimpy, even

WHAT INCREASES APPETITE, WHAT HELPS YOU CONTROL IT

FACTORS THAT MAKE YOU HUNGRY

▶ **An empty stomach:** Alerted to your need for energy by a hormone produced in your stomach, your brain tells you it's time to eat.

▶ **The sight and smell of food:** You've heard of Pavlov's dogs, who were conditioned to salivate as soon as they saw or heard the bell of the assistant who fed them. Humans also have a learned response to food.

▶ **Eating:** Eating alerts your brain to the presence of food, and that makes you want to eat even more.

▶ **Defending your set point:** When your body weight dips below the range your genetics dictate it should be, hormonal activity conspires to increase your appetite.

▶ **A need to cope with stress or emotional issues:** Knowing that food can calm you and desensitize you to pain or discomfort makes you crave it in times of need.

FACTORS THAT HELP CONTROL APPETITE

▶ **Eating regular meals and snacks:** If you eat consistently, approximately every three to four hours, your blood sugar level won't have the opportunity to drop so low that you get to the point of feeling famished and out of control.

▶ **Eating well-balanced meals and snacks:** Consuming a combination of protein, fat, and fiber-rich carbohydrates can buy you an extra hour of satiety.

▶ **Getting enough calories:** A green salad with a little dressing isn't enough of a meal. Make sure you're not undereating; you'll get hungry again right away.

▶ **Resolving emotional issues:** Examining and remedying the underlying causes of emotional hunger will help you stop turning to food for comfort.

▶ **Distraction and fulfillment:** If you spend your time doing other things that make you feel good, you're going to feel less of a need to eat.

▶ **A diet packed with high-fiber and water-rich foods:** Foods that slow down digestion help your blood sugar level stay steady and keep you satisfied longer. Bulky foods with fewer calories per gram help satisfy your need for volume at a low-calorie cost.

▶ **Physical activity:** If you're new to exercise or increasing your workout intensity markedly, you may experience an increase in your appetite at first, but not so much that the calories you take in will end up being more than those you burn off. One study seems to indicate this may be especially true if you exercise fifteen to thirty minutes before you eat a meal.

▶ **Following the hunger scale:** Eating only when you're at a 3 or 4 on the hunger scale and stopping when you hit 5 or 6 will help you tune into what's real hunger and real satisfaction so that you don't just eat out of habit (see page 92).

▶ **Waiting twenty minutes before deciding whether to continue eating:** That's how long it takes your brain to receive fullness signals. In the meantime, your appetite may be like a runaway train. Putting on the brakes for a while and allowing your brain to catch up with your body almost always leads to the decision to not eat any more.

▶ **A good night's sleep:** Getting enough shut-eye helps prevent any disruption of the hormones that control appetite.

if your stomach says differently. As you go from being a big-portion eater to someone who's satisfied with more moderate amounts, high-fiber and water-rich foods are going to help you make the transition. These foods will let you eat more (think of a big bowl of hearty vegetable soup versus a small cup of cream of broccoli, both of which may have the same amount of calories), feel less hungry, and keep your calorie intake in check.

I want to point out that all the recommended meals and many of the snacks in the Best Life Diet contain a mixture of carbohydrates, protein, and fat. This is because eating all three of these nutrients together seems to be more satisfying than eating any of them alone; each brings something to the table. Protein may be the most satiating. Many studies show that people feel more satisfied and eat fewer calories later on after having meals rich in protein. Scientists aren't sure why protein is so satiating, but theorize that it may affect hormones that supress the appetite. Carbohydrates have bulk; they expand your stomach and activate the nerves in the stomach lining that tell your brain to stop eating. They also raise your blood sugar level, providing both immediate and long-term energy. Fat's role is to slow down digestion, delaying the time before your stomach becomes empty and begins signaling your brain to eat again. Together, protein, carbohydrates, and fat are going to maximize how full you feel on the fewest number of calories.

And how full should you feel? In the section of this phase devoted to the hunger scale, you're going to learn some ways to analyze your hunger. Getting better at listening to your body and making a conscious effort to pause before you decide to eat a second helping or dessert is going to allow you to manage your appetite better. Hunger, or, more precisely, what you *perceive* to be hunger, can often be nothing more than habit. As you learn to eat more mindfully, it's a habit that's going to become easier to break.

There's one last element of appetite control that I want to mention that may surprise you: sleep. There is increasing evidence that the amount and quality of sleep you get may affect your body weight (and not because tossing and turning burns calories!). Scientists are finding that lack of sleep disrupts the balance of ghrelin and leptin, the hunger on and off switches, and that people who are sleep-deprived have increased appetites. The more we learn about the body, the more indication there is that all healthy habits are connected. Now we know that getting a good night's sleep and maintaining a healthy body weight are linked, too.

Understand the Emotional Reasons for Your Hunger

Feeling the urge to eat though you're not physically hungry. Still feeling pangs of hunger despite the fact that you've just eaten enough to feed a linebacker. Eating in secret. Feeling guilty about what and how much you eat. Running out to the store at 10 P.M. to satisfy a craving. Declining social invitations so you can stay home and eat. Feeling panicky when your favorite food is out of stock. If you're an emotional eater, these are things you've probably experienced at one time or another. There may be a hole somewhere in your life, and you're trying to fill it with food.

Although emotions don't necessarily trigger the same physiological chain of reactions that an empty stomach does, your body can experience some very real cravings that originate from the reward centers of the brain. When you eat for comfort, food does its job: it soothes and calms you. Within the circuitry of your brain, this reinforces food's desirability, and it makes you want more of it. This pattern is much like drug addiction; however, unlike drugs, which you can live without, food is essential to your survival. What's more, food is readily available, relatively inexpensive, and a far more socially acceptable coping tool than drugs or alcohol. Food may make you feel good, but if you have other things in your life that also make you feel good (and fewer things that make you feel bad), you're not going to feel such a strong need to overeat.

Eating too much is often a symptom of something else that may be wrong in your life. When you discover what that something is, as I urged you to begin doing in the chapter "Understanding Your Weight," you can work toward changing it, and *that*—along with ending overeating and subsequently losing weight—is going to move you toward your best life.

Discovering the emotional reasons you overeat, then mending the problems behind them takes time. The self-discovery process that you began at the outset of this program is a good start, but you can get even greater insight by using the exercise called the Circle of Life, which I mentioned earlier in the book. I'd like to introduce you to the basic premise.

The point of this exercise is to help you explore all the areas of your life and determine which, if any, are problematic or unfulfilled and in need of your attention. Begin by writing down all the elements you consider part of a fulfilled life. Some common ones might be family, romance, friends, career, community, spirituality, physical health, financial health, hobbies, and other personal interests. Now go down the list and put a plus or minus next to each element, depending on how well it's going in your life. A plus means you have few or no complaints; a minus means you're disappointed in the way things are going. The elements that are associated with minuses are really what you need to pay particular attention to—they're probably the areas of your life that you're going to need to address if you hope to get to the root of your overeating.

As part of your efforts to examine and recognize what's causing your emotional eating, it's also a good idea to explore the ideas you have about yourself and your capabilities. One of the greatest barriers to weight loss is a deep-seated belief that you're either not deserving or not worthy of happiness or success. That may sound crazy—why would you have put so much effort into losing weight if you didn't really want to lose weight or believe that you could do it?—but I see it all the time. Many people are undermined by deeply buried emotions and insecurities that hark all the way back to childhood. Not everyone is hampered by self-doubt of this kind, but it's definitely worth exploring. As you're checking in on all the different areas of your life, check in on your feelings about success, too. Are you open to it? And if not, why?

Entering into a weight-loss program means that you have to give yourself the time and attention you deserve. This is not to say that you should shirk your responsibilities to others, but you really have to take a stand and do what's right for *you*. I have had many clients who felt they needed to eat unhealthy foods and more food than they really wanted just to keep the people around them happy. They'd make and eat meals that were fattening or bring home greasy take-out because their family "demanded" it. Or they'd go out with friends for drinks, high-calorie meals, or desserts because they didn't want to be a party pooper. But in the end, by not doing what was best for themselves, they weren't doing their family and friends any favors, either. To be happy and the kind of person others want to be around, you need to attend to your own well-being. It may feel great to go along with the crowd for a while, but ultimately you're going to start to feel sad and/or resentful about not controlling your own life.

Not too long ago, I was contacted by an American woman living in Australia, where she'd moved to live with her husband, who was Australian. She had come home for a visit to see her family and was upset by some jokes that her brother had made about her weight. It was true that she had gained about 20 pounds in the year that she'd been living away from home, and her brother's jokes, though cruel, made her face up to the fact that her weight had gotten out of control. We talked for a while, and eventually she admitted that she didn't like living in Australia and missed her friends and family back home. But she was crazy about her husband and wanted him to be happy, so she was keeping mum about her discontent. It was obvious to me that ignoring her own interests had led her to use food to buffer her feelings of sadness and loneliness. I sent her back to Australia with an assignment: to be honest about her feelings with her husband and try to find things in Australia that would improve how she felt about living there.

The next time I heard from the woman, she had lost almost all her excess weight. She had found a job that she really loved and that made her feel more a part of the community. She didn't feel the need to turn to food so much anymore, and now that she was busier, she didn't have much opportunity to overeat, either.

People gain weight for different reasons, and they fail to lose weight or keep it off for different reasons, too. One common reason is that extra pounds, even if they feel unwanted, provide a certain amount of security. Every time you look in the mirror, perhaps you are unhappy with what you see, but subconsciously you may feel very well protected. Because of this, as soon as the pounds start to roll off, you may begin to feel vulnerable, and subsequently, ambivalent about the results of your efforts. You're losing your armor: the excess weight you hide behind so that you don't have to deal with things like your relationships with other people, your sexuality, or the expectations of your family and friends. Inevitably, when you start to lose weight, people are going to notice that you've changed; they're going to pay attention to you, and suddenly you may have to confront many issues and situations that you've been avoiding.

I can see how that can be daunting, but don't let it hinder you. As Oprah said in her foreword, it's only when you peel back the layers and let yourself become more exposed that you can really be free: "free to work out, free to eat responsibly, free to live the life you want and deserve to live." Take the steps to change your life; you'll lose weight, *and* a great weight will be lifted off your shoulders.

ELIMINATING EMOTIONAL EATING STEP-BY-STEP

I've said before that I don't expect you to change your life overnight, and you shouldn't expect it of yourself. But that doesn't mean you shouldn't start working on it right now. Try and do at least one small thing every day to improve each area of your life. That could mean that you pick up the phone, send an email, or write a letter; meditate; say a prayer; or read a book. Maybe it's just carving out fifteen minutes for yourself every night to do something physically pleasurable, like taking a bath or stretching your muscles. Maybe it's taking an even bigger step such as making an appointment with a couples therapist or asserting yourself with your kids. But make a point of doing *something.* As you concentrate on balancing your meals, simultaneously endeavor to balance your life. Work toward making your voice heard in relationships and strengthening your connections with others. Ask yourself what you want in this world, and go after it in every way you can.

Everybody needs something to make them feel good, and ultimately, when you feel good about your life, you're going to stop eating for emotional sustenance. But don't wait until you resolve everything in your life perfectly before allowing yourself to take pleasure in your accomplishments. Take pleasure in the process of moving your life forward. Allow yourself to take satisfaction in your efforts every day that you take another small step toward improving your well-being. Each of those small steps is going to get you closer to your goal, and being able to feel good about the direction you're going in is going to motivate you to stick with it until you reach the end.

Also keep in mind that other things can "feed" your brain's hunger to be soothed and calmed besides food. It's not a bad thing to want comfort; it's actually a healthy impulse to want to drive away the doldrums. However, it's very important to realize that eating is not your only option. Exercise is a powerful substitute—its ability to improve one's mood is well documented, and taking a walk or popping in a workout DVD is a great way to activate mood-elevating endorphins. But anything you love doing— talking to friends, listening to music, reading a book, working on an art project, making a scrapbook, taking part in a book group, writing in your journal, perusing travel guides as you dream about a future vacation, knitting, sewing, playing cards or board games, doing crossword puzzles—can also substitute for a bag of tortilla chips or carton of ice cream. You just need to make a conscious effort to choose these pursuits over food. If you're used to running to the refrigerator when you're sad or angry, bored or lonely, depressed or anxious, you need to pause and ask yourself what else you can do.

I do want to qualify this by saying that it can take some time before you feel that engaging in other things is as pleasurable as eating. The trail to your refrigerator is not the only pathway that is well trodden: the neurocircuitry pathways in your brain are also well worn. Because you're used to getting your pleasure from food, you essentially need to retrain your brain and create new pathways so that you derive as much (or even more) enjoyment from other types of fulfilling activities. After a while, though, you will adapt to the change and won't miss the cake and candy. Ultimately, you'll get much greater, deeper satisfaction out of those life-improving alternatives.

MINDLESS EATING

Sometimes you may eat because your physical hunger is so insistent that you can't ignore it. Sometimes you may eat because you need relief from stress or the negative emotions you're experiencing. I'm willing to bet that you also sometimes eat for absolutely no reason at all other than you're used to doing so whether or not you're even hungry. Sitting in front of the television with a bowl of trail mix. Gobbling down M&M's while you work at your desk. Nibbling on pretzels at your kid's soccer game. Passing around a big bag of cheese puffs in the car. This is mindless eating.

A lot of people not only don't pay attention to their own internal cues, but they also depend on cues outside themselves to tell them when they should stop eating. A study conducted at the University of Illinois at Urbana–Champaign, for instance, found that many students decided to put down their forks or glasses only when everyone else was finished, when they ran out of a beverage, when it was getting late, when others thought it was normal to stop, when they finished reading, or when the TV show they were watching was over. I wasn't surprised to learn that the people who paid the most attention to external cues were also the people who weighed the most.

You'll do away with a lot of mindless eating when you begin using the hunger scale (page 92), but it's also important to give eating your full attention. Don't eat while you're doing things other than enjoying the company of friends and family. If you're eating alone, don't do it while reading a magazine or watching TV; these are distractions that will prevent you from monitoring your hunger and experiencing the pleasure of eating. If you absentmindedly wolf down a sandwich, you're going to end up noticing that the sandwich is suddenly gone but you don't feel like you've really eaten. Then what are you going to do? Eat some more.

So here are some eating rules to live by: Eat out of hunger, not habit. Savor your food; eat slowly and pay attention to what you're eating. Know when to stop eating by gauging your hunger instead of depending on cues from your environment (such as everyone else at the table being done). Eat mindfully, and you'll eat considerably less and fully experience the pleasure of eating.

Use the Hunger Scale

I've talked about true physical hunger, emotional hunger, and the difference between the two. I think it's important to know about both so that you can understand the reasons why you eat and work on limiting your emotional eating. But when it comes down to the decisions about how much you should eat, what you should eat, and if in fact you should eat anything at all, it doesn't really matter *why* you're hungry. What matters is that you have a strategy in place to help you handle your appetite, whatever the cause.

I've already mentioned several of them (see the box on pages 82–83 for a rundown on all the things that will help you control your hunger), and now I'd like to add the most important strategy to the group: using the hunger scale. This tool for gauging how hungry you feel is going to help you set some limits and avoid eating mindlessly. When you use it properly, the hunger scale allows you to get feedback from your body so that you know when to stop eating. Personally, I think most people don't need to count calories or measure portion sizes if they're very in touch with their hunger. That's what this scale is going to help you accomplish.

The hunger scale is a ten-point scale (see page 92) based on different stages of physical fullness (or emptiness, as the case may be). Nutritionists have used it for years to help clients have an inner dialogue with themselves when they feel the need to eat. Eating is so often a reflexive act: you feel a bit of hunger, so you eat, never stopping to ask yourself, "How hungry am I *really*? Do I actually need to eat?" The beauty of the hunger scale is that it gives you some guidelines to go by and lets you see that hunger isn't just hunger—there are times when you actually do need to eat and times when you can get by without doing it.

More than anything, though, the hunger scale is going to help you avoid the peaks and valleys of hunger; you're not going to feel stuffed, and you're not going to be ravenous. That, in turn, is going to lead to smarter, more mindful eating, and as a result, less body fat. The scale is easy to use, although it may feel awkward at first. After a while, you're not even going to have to think about it; cutting off your eating at the appropriate time will just come naturally.

Basically, the hunger scale helps you answer two questions: "Do I need to eat?" and, when you're already eating, "Should I eat more?" Your hunger level when you begin eating should be 3 or 4. You're just starting to get hungry, or maybe you're feeling a bit uncomfortable. While you may not always be at a 3 or 4 when it's mealtime, and at breakfast you may not feel hungry at all, it's important to adhere to the three-meals-a-day guideline anyway. If you're not at the point yet where you're automatically waking up hungry, go ahead and eat breakfast whether you've worked up to a 3 or not. Don't, however, force a snack. If you're not at a 3 or 4, save the snack for when you're actually hungry.

What you don't want to do at any time of the day is fall *below* a 3 or 4, because that means you've waited too long to eat, and that can make you vulnerable to overeating. Whenever you go to the table feeling starved, you're going to want to eat anything and everything in sight, and it's especially hard to rein in your impulses when you're feeling weak and tired.

During this phase of aggressive weight loss, when you're already eating a meal or snack you should stop eating when you get to a 5 on the hunger scale. A 5 is the point at which you can be confident that you are eating a little less than your body is burning. At 5 you're not really still hungry, but you're not really full, an indication that you are undereating slightly (though not enough to put you in danger of overeating later on). Later in this program, when you have met your weight-loss goals and are maintaining your weight, you can stop eating at level 6 on the scale, which will allow you to raise your calorie intake a bit. When you're at a 6, you know the calories you take in are pretty much in line with the calories you burn; you're breaking even. Keep in mind that whether you're in a losing or a maintaining phase, you don't ever want to hit the point where you feel even a tiny bit uncomfortable: satisfied, yes; uncomfortable, no.

One reason constantly monitoring your hunger is important is because, in some ways, eating turns the body into a runaway train bent on consuming more and more. Eating actually triggers the release of chemicals in the body that encourage you to keep going, at least for a little while. It's another throwback to the days when humans needed to eat all that they could while it was available. Another reason to keep on top of your hunger is because it takes some time for digestion to occur and for your blood sugar to rise after you eat. Before you make the decision to have a second helping or dessert, pause for fifteen to twenty minutes. There is always a lag time between eating and feelings of satisfaction, and that's why it's critical to make a conscious effort to put on the brakes, at least for a while. You probably won't need to eat more. So leave the table, go for a walk, do something else, and then check in with yourself again to see where you are on the hunger scale. If you're in a restaurant, suggest going somewhere else for dessert. By the time you get there, chances are you're going to get the message that you've had enough and call it a night. *The pause is one of the most important tools in your arsenal! It's going to be your key to substantial weight loss.*

The great thing about using the hunger scale now is that after you've used it for a while, knowing when to stop eating is going to become almost second nature. It will still be a conscious act, but not one you have to think much about.

THE HUNGER SCALE

10 Stuffed: You are so full, you feel nauseous.

9 Very uncomfortably full: You need to loosen your clothes.

8 Uncomfortably full: You feel bloated.

7 Full: You feel a little bit uncomfortable.

6 Perfectly comfortable: You feel satisfied.

5 Comfortable: You're more or less satisfied, but could eat a little more.

4 Slightly uncomfortable: You're just beginning to feel signs of hunger.

3 Uncomfortable: Your stomach is rumbling.

2 Very uncomfortable: You feel irritable and unable to concentrate.

1 Weak and light-headed: Your stomach acid is churning.

For now, though, the scale is going to help you get through the day without eating too much or letting yourself get dangerously hungry. When you're doing everything right, I think you'll be surprised at how manageable your hunger seems. You're not going to have those highs where you're so full that you feel nauseous and guilty or those lows that lead you to overeat to the point of feeling nauseous and guilty (as you can see, it's a vicious cycle). Using the hunger scale will also help you judge if you're where you want to be when you're ready for bed at night. In Phase One, I explained that the eating cutoff time (at least two hours before sleeping) ensures that you turn in feeling a slight tug of hunger. Now let's put a hunger scale number on it: 4. When your body signals you that it needs food, even if the signal is just a whisper, and you don't answer the call, it's going to turn to your stored fat for fuel. That's what you want to happen. Every time it does, you're losing body fat.

Like everything you're doing during this phase, getting a real feel for the hunger scale may take some time. On occasion you may feel that even if the number you're at on the scale doesn't permit it, the urge to eat is strong and hard to resist. When this occurs, I suggest that you occupy yourself with something that you enjoy doing other than eating. One effective technique is to make yourself a cup of tea and pull out your journal, and use this time to write about any topic of interest to you, especially ways to improve your life. Distract yourself and you're likely to forget all about your urge to eat.

DIETARY CHANGES

A Note About Adding More Structure
to Your Diet If You Like

I'm not a big believer in living your life by numbers; that is, I don't think you should have to spend your days and nights counting calories. While it may help some people to count calories, I don't think it's necessary in order to succeed on this program. In my experience, the vast majority of the people who get themselves moving, follow the meal-structuring and cutoff time guidelines in Phase One, gauge their hunger, watch their portions, and remove a few unhealthy (and high-calorie) foods from their diets lose a significant number of pounds—and all without counting calories.

That said, it's still a good idea to be generally aware of calories so when you check package labels and the calories on recipes, you'll have a sense of whether those foods fit into a moderate eating plan. Plus, in Phase Three, you'll be getting Anything Goes calories to spend on foods you like, so you do need to have *some* concept of how much you're eating.

It may be helpful to you to take a look at the Best Life Diet Guidelines starting on page 124. This guide lets you know how many servings of each type of food (and about how many calories) you should be eating according to how much activity you do each week. It also provides information on what's considered a serving, which can help you keep your portions down to size. It's a helpful guide, though ultimately, for most people, being in tune with your hunger is the best way to monitor how much you eat. Also take a look at the Best Life Diet Meal Plans (page 167–190). These menus incorporate the appropriate amount of servings for your activity level. If you don't want to worry about how many servings of this and that you should be eating, you don't have to; all the work is already done for you. Following these meal plans isn't required for success in this program; they're simply there to give you some ideas about what to eat and to provide you with a snapshot of what a healthy diet looks like. Check out "Oprah's Seven-Day Food Diary" on pages 161–167 and you can get a peek into how Oprah has used the principles of the Best Life Diet in her life.

As I said earlier, the vast majority of people can do very well just using the hunger scale to help them figure out what their calorie intake should be, but there are also some people who will find the Best Life Diet Guidelines, What's a Serving? *and* the Best Life Diet Meal Plans (pages 124, 126, 167) both useful and necessary. Some physical conditions simply make it harder to lose weight, and if you have one of them, you may need to adhere tightly to a specific calorie level to achieve success. People who have diabetes or certain thyroid conditions or who are insulin resistant, post-menopausal, or on medications that alter appetite or the metabolism usually have to be more meticulous about what they eat. Likewise, people whose genetics cause them to stubbornly cling to body fat or who have trouble losing weight now because they've lost and gained it so many times throughout the years may need to stay within a very narrow calorie range to shed pounds successfully. If you fall into any of these categories or just have a particularly hard time losing weight, these guidelines will be of great value.

You may also want to use this information if you simply do better with more structure. Maybe you tend to have more success when you have stricter guidelines about how much and what to eat. Maybe you've only ever lost weight while sticking to calorie rules and meal plans, and you've not only come to expect them, but you're also slightly fearful of approaching weight loss without them. Then by all means, use the serving guidelines and meal plans. But you could also just try to follow all the objectives I've laid out for you in this phase and see how you do without using them. If you're not losing weight, you can always change course and use them.

In truth, no weight-loss program can tell you the exact number of calories you need to eat to lose weight unless it's interactive. When I work with clients one-on-one, I can give them a good sense of the number of calories they need to eat because I know their personal habits and limitations, and I'm getting feedback from them all the time. I can see their progress and make adjustments accordingly. With the Best Life Diet Guidelines and Best Life Diet Meal Plans, I have tried to present calorie ranges that will work for *most* people given their activity level. Taking activity as well as gender into account when devising these guidelines makes them different and, I think, a cut above the one-size-fits-all diets. It may still take some trial and error to fine-tune your calorie counts, but for most people, the Best Life guidelines will be accurate.

If you want to take fine-tuning this diet to your specific needs even further, you have the opportunity to do so at www.thebestlife.com. There you can get the Best Life Diet, including additional detailed weekly meal plans modified for lowering cholesterol or for food allergies; a version without red meat; and one that's lacto-ovo vegetarian. If you require more structure or are dealing with some particular limitations, this is a great way to ensure that you get all the support you need.

Even if you prefer having a particular calorie count to stick to and like having menu plans to follow, there will likely come a time when you become so familiar with what constitutes your particular Best Life Diet that you no longer need to think about calories and menus. My goal is to get you to a point where healthy eating just comes naturally to you. You'll instinctively know how to divide up your calories during the day and practically be able to put together a nutritious, reasonably proportioned meal with your eyes closed. You'll know you're living your best life when the details of eating well no longer weigh heavily on your mind.

Eat Reasonable Portions

One way that you're going to lower your calorie intake so that you lose a significant number of pounds during this phase is to pare down your portion sizes. Reasonable portions are the key to getting calories under control, but don't be surprised if you don't know what constitutes a reasonable portion. In these days of super-sized bowls of pasta and burritos you need to hold with two hands, it's hard to tell what an appropriate serving is. There's no doubt that restaurant portion sizes have increased exponentially since the 1980s, and they're larger than what's considered healthy. Researchers at New York University have noted that many fast-food items are now two to five times larger than their original incarnations. Even cookie recipes in cookbooks have been changed so that they produce larger cookies than they used to.

While there are many theories as to why obesity rates have jumped so high in the last few decades, it doesn't seem to be a coincidence that the increase in portion sizes has risen in tandem with the increase in body fat. That's a good indication to me that no weight-loss program can succeed without attention to portion control.

It would help if all restaurants and food manufacturers simply produced and served food in sensible portions. They are, though, somewhat caught between a rock and a hard place. On the one hand, they're doing a disservice to us all by creating wildly big serving sizes. On the other hand, they're also answering a demand. Americans like to get a big bang for their buck and aren't afraid to take their business elsewhere if they don't get it. People have come to expect oversize portions, and those in the business of supplying food feel compelled by economics to comply.

That may be why buffets seem to be so popular, but I have to confess that I don't see the allure. Buffets are calorie traps. When you're confronted with mountains of food—and all at one price—it's hard not to feel obligated to put as much on your plate as possible. And you feel like you've got to clean that plate, too, because what sense would it make to go to a buffet if you couldn't go back for more? If you've ever made it through a buffet without overeating, I congratulate you! I also don't like buffets for other reasons. Sneeze guards or no sneeze guards, the food on buffet tables seems like prime real estate for germs and bacteria. Add to that the fact that the food usually isn't very fresh-tasting or kept at an appealing temperature, and you've lost me. Make controlling your portions easier by staying away from buffets.

While buffets probably aren't going away anytime soon, there has been somewhat of a backlash against the super-sizing of food, and several food companies and restaurants are taking note. In fact, some food manufacturers are now selling snacks in 100-calorie packages, and many companies have also put more realistic serving sizes on the nutrition panels of their products. These are trends that I hope will continue to catch on, because they're going to make it easier to control your intake and get the information you need to help you figure out, given the calorie count you're aiming for, how much of a food you should eat.

There is, though, no substitute for your own vigilance when it comes to portion control. The easiest way to judge whether or not you're consuming reasonable portions is to use your hunger-scale smarts. When you're consistent about gauging your hunger, you'll be able to tell if you are eating too much as well as if you're eating too little. Ceasing to eat when you hit 5 on the scale is the key to keeping your calories at a level that will cause weight loss; ceasing to eat when you hit 6 will keep your calories at the break-even point for maintenance. Practice this technique over and over again, and pretty soon it's going to become automatic. You're going to *know* how much you should and shouldn't eat, just by looking at your food.

This is important, because you can't always rely on food manufacturers or restaurants to dish out moderate portions. It's the rare restaurant that's going to serve you a steak that's a reasonably sized portion; you're the one who has to put on the brakes by either sharing the steak or taking whatever's left once you hit level 5 home in a doggy bag. You've also got to get over the idea that bigger is better because it may save you money. Just because you can get double the popcorn for just a quarter more at the movies doesn't mean that you should buy it. You may get a deal at the concession stand, but what about the money you're going to have to invest in healthcare because you opted for the bigger size over and over again? The super-sized deal isn't worth it.

If you still feel you need some backup to ensure you're eating moderate portions, you can turn to two charts in this book: What's a Serving?, on page 126, and the serving guidelines on page 125. The first chart gives you a rundown of what is considered a reasonable serving in every food group; the second tells you how many servings you should get per day based on your gender and activity level. Let those be your guide to eating moderately.

Shaving down the size of your servings is going to bring about substantial weight loss, especially if you have always subscribed to "the bigger, the better" way of thinking. Like any significant change, paring down is going to take some getting used to. You not only have to adjust your stomach to getting less food, but you also have to adjust your eye. Since you're used to seeing more food on the plate, your brain is going to register "skimpy" when you cut portions down in size. But your brain will adapt. To help it along, use smaller plates and bowls so servings will look bigger; it's an old trick, but one that really works.

Remove Six Unhealthy Foods from Your Diet

You're now at the point where I want you to start taking a critical look at the food you're eating and making some changes. It's a little like going through your bookshelves and weeding out the volumes you don't want or need anymore. You not only get rid of what's unnecessary, but you also free up space to put new books on your shelves. Here you'll be eliminating a few foods that are detrimental to your health and weight-loss efforts while freeing up space in your diet for those that will enhance your well-being.

Before I get to the specifics, I want to talk a little bit about the kinds of foods out there in today's marketplace. Right now there's a lot of debate about how much responsibility food companies should bear for public health. As a result, many manufacturers are trying harder to produce more nutritious products, and I'm thrilled about it. I see it as a really positive step forward. But I also think that, just as it's each individual's job to be vigilant about portion sizes, it's also each person's responsibility to pay close attention to what he or she buys and eats. Get as much information about the food you consume as possible so that you don't fall into the trap of assuming that something is healthy when in fact it's nothing of the sort.

The priority of people who package and distribute food is to sell their products, and they know that if their products don't taste good, then you won't buy them. Food companies also want to answer our health concerns, not necessarily out of the goodness of their hearts (though some companies truly are conscientious), but because this, too, influences their bottom line. They're trying to walk a fine line; if they change a product too much to make it healthier, there's a good chance you'll walk away from it. Yet as we get more educated about nutrition and get wise to the fact that a food contains something that threatens our health, we're also likely to stop buying that food. I give my blessing to many different products when I believe the companies behind them have found that all-important balance between good taste and good health. The products on which you'll find the Best Life seal of approval are excellent sources of nutrients while low enough in calories to help you control your weight. Plus, you can find them at any supermarket.

And while I'm on the subject of supermarkets, I want to mention that they are where you can make or break your weight-loss goals. It's there that you'll choose products that will support your efforts or derail them, where you decide whether you're going to be successful or not. I check out every product that I buy, and I urge you to do so as well. It's critical that you also carefully scrutinize every food you put in your grocery cart. That means becoming an avid reader of the ingredient list and nutrition panel on a product, and when there are none—if you're buying prepared food, from a farmer's market, or from a roadside stand—that you ask the seller as many questions as possible. It's not enough to read the front of the label on a product, because, frankly, many labels are misleading. You've got to check out the fine print, too.

I'll give you an example. A client of mine bought organic peanut butter, figuring it was the healthiest option on the shelf. When she tasted the peanut butter, she thought it seemed kind of sweet, so she looked at the back of the jar to see if anything had been added to it. Much to her surprise, the ingredients listed high-fructose corn syrup along with the peanuts and salt. Because the product was labeled organic, she just assumed it didn't contain nonessential ingredients like high-fructose corn syrup (and peanut butter, at least in my opinion, is one of those foods that really don't need anything extra). I can't stress this enough: *Always read the ingredients list.*

The good news is that, in most cases, it really is possible to find out what's in the food you're buying. It may require doing a little more legwork (some chain restaurants list nutrition information on their websites) and asking questions of not-always-happy-to-answer restaurant employees, but it's well worth your time, and it can be the difference between success and failure on a weight-loss program. Whenever possible, know what you're eating, and check my website frequently. I'm going to be constantly updating it with new foods and beverages that comply with the Best Life guidelines.

During this phase of the Best Life Diet, you need to start being particularly vigilant about removing these six foods: soda, foods that contain trans fats, fried foods, white bread, and high-fat milk and yogurt products. When you consider that there are thousands of foods out there and that you only have to concern yourself with six of them right now, this should feel like a fairly simple task. But as simple it may seem, it's going to help you cut calories dramatically, particularly if you're a big soda drinker. Here's what you need to know about each of the six foods and what you should replace them with.

SODA (POP)

In Phase One, I urged you to drink water not only to keep you adequately hydrated, but also in the hope that if you were drinking plenty of water, you wouldn't feel the need to drink sugary sodas. Well, if you're still drinking soda, cut it out! Seriously, soda is a major problem for anyone trying to lose weight (and I'd add that it's a health problem for anyone *not* trying to lose weight, too). It's probably the number one source of empty calories, and by that I mean it's a food that has plenty of calories but doesn't provide any nutrients. It's nutritionally bankrupt. Recently, a USDA researcher found that for two-thirds of Americans, soda provides more of their daily calories than any other food. She also found the obesity rate is higher among those soda-drinking Americans. New research has shown that by drinking just one twelve-ounce soda a day, you can gain 15 pounds in one year. Other studies have shown that women who drink one or more sugary sodas a day are more prone to diabetes.

It gets worse: A recent study found that drinking as little as one soda daily is associated with a 50 percent increased risk of developing metabolic syndrome. Metabolic syndrome is a cluster of conditions that contribute to heart disease. The conditions include high blood sugar, high blood pressure, high levels of a blood fat called triglycerides, low levels of HDL (the "good" cholesterol), and a large waistline (35 inches or more for women, 40 inches or more for men). What's particularly surprising—and alarming—about this study is that diet soda was just as risky as regular. Researchers aren't sure why diet drinks are also harmful, but speculate that they may set people up to eat more sweets. Another theory is that an ingredient in many soft drinks—caramel—may promote glycation products,

sugar/protein clusters linked to insulin resistance (the first step to diabetes) and inflammation (a risk factor for heart disease and other ills). The
research, sponsored by the National Heart, Lung, and Blood Institute,
looked at soft drink comsumption in men and women who are part of the
long-running Framingham Heart Study, in Framingham Massachusetts.

And here's what I've observed about diet soda: many people end up
compensating, or even *over*compensating, for the absent calories because
they consciously or unconsciously feel that drinking a no-cal beverage gives
them extra latitude to eat. I can't tell you how many times I've stood in line
behind someone at the store buying candy, cookies, and a diet drink, or
watched someone at a restaurant order a piece of pie and a diet soda. So
be careful: eliminating calories in one place doesn't necessarily mean you
should make them up elsewhere.

So should you give up diet soda as well? Here's what I think about artificially sweetened sodas: If you feel very attached to these drinks and they
help you to lose weight, then continue to drink them—*in moderation*. But I
also recommend that you wean yourself off them, or at least try to get down
to one a day, because if you drink a lot of diet soda, you're never going to
lose your taste for super-sweet food. Part of the Best Life Diet program is to
get you to change your taste preferences so that you feel less of a desire for
the super-sweet, super-fatty and super-salty tastes that are the hallmark of
highly processed junk food. Drinking artificially sweetened soda, some of
which are even sweeter-tasting than sugar-sweetened sodas, can perpetuate
your desire for that intense flavor. Plus, there are now so many great low- or
no-calorie alternatives to diet soda on the market and more on the way.

What to Drink Instead: Water, Milk, Juice, Tea Water, plain or flavored,
you're probably not surprised to hear, is my first choice as a soda substitute.
But there are other beverages I recommend, too. Skim milk, 1 percent
milk, or calcium-enriched soymilk are good choices. Fruit juice is another,
but with a qualification: although it has plenty of the nutrients you need,
juice is just as high in calories as soda, so consume it in moderation and as
it fits into your calorie guidelines. Try to limit yourself to one glass per day,
or cut it with soda water to make a sparkler. Also be sure to choose pure
fruit juices instead of fruit *drinks,* which are bolstered with sweeteners. My
personal favorite fruit juice is grapefruit; it's not too sweet and it's loaded

with disease-fighting phytonutrients. Calcium-enriched orange, tangerine, and pomegranate juices are also good choices.

Another good beverage choice is iced tea. I love teas because they come in so many flavors as well as decaffeinated and herbal varieties. I love herbal teas for their soothing quality and lack of caffeine, but teas made from green or black leaves have been shown to have substantial health benefits. Black tea seems to lower the risk of heart disease and stroke, while green and black teas both appear to boost the immune system and protect against some forms of cancer. If you buy bottled iced tea, look for unsweetened varieties. One I like that you might try is Lipton's unsweetened tea, which is widely available in stores.

FOODS WITH TRANS FATS

I put trans-fatty acids on my hit list not only because foods high in trans fats—like some cookies, French fries, and microwave popcorn—are usually high in calories, but also because trans fats can be a threat to your health. It's now clear that trans fats are even more artery-clogging than saturated fat (which is found primarily in animal foods). Not only do they raise LDL ("bad") cholesterol, but they also lower HDL ("good") cholesterol. Some preliminary research now also suggests that you may be more likely to gain weight if you eat trans fats than if you eat healthy monounsaturated fats (like olive oil), even if you consume the same amount of calories of both. It may be that a calorie is not a calorie after all. What's more, trans fats may also cause body fat to be stored in the abdominal area, a serious health concern because abdominal fat is associated with a greater risk of heart disease.

Trans fats are created by adding hydrogen to vegetable oil, a process that solidifies the oil and makes it more stable. This process is called partial hydrogenation, and *partially hydrogenated* vegetable oils are the ingredient on the label that's going to tell you whether or not a food contains trans fats. Margarine and vegetable shortenings are two of the biggest sources of trans fats, though you can now also find varieties labeled "0 grams trans fat" on the market. Frozen meals, crackers, ramen soups, cake mixes, nondairy creamers, chips, candy, and fried food (which I'll get to next) tend to be the biggest trans fat offenders.

What's not commonly known is that trans fat also occurs naturally in dairy and meat: the higher the fat content of these foods, the higher the levels. For instance, nonfat milk has no trans fat; whole milk has about 0.2 g per cup. High-fat meats have about 1.1 g per four ounces. (The maximum amount of trans fat you should get per day is described at the end of this section.) So making the choices encouraged on this program—lean meats and 1 percent or nonfat dairy—means you're getting virtually no trans fat. Interestingly, the type of trans fat in dairy and meat is slightly different chemically from the artificially created fat. While research comparing the health effects of the two is still sparse, it's indicating that natural trans fat may not be bad for the heart.

Other sources of trans fat, though minor ones, are regular oils found in the supermarket. The trans fat is formed when these oils are heated and refined. It's unclear how much trans fat is in these oils, but experts believe it's in the ballpark of 3 percent or less of total fat. So it appears that the levels in these oils are so negligible that they don't pose a health hazard.

You may have noticed hydrogenated oil (as opposed to partially hydrogenated oil) on ingredient lists. It's the same chemical process, but taken a step further, and no trans fats are produced. But depending on the oil used, it could be high in unhealthy saturated fat.

Besides checking a product's ingredients to see if partially hydrogenated vegetable oil is listed, you can determine whether a food contains a substantial amount of trans fats by reading the nutrition facts panel. The FDA has now mandated that trans fat content be included in the panel of any processed food. There is one little technicality, though, that can make the information confusing. A food may contain partially hydrogenated vegetable oil, but if the amount is negligible—0.49 g or less—the FDA still allows the manufacturer to say the food has 0 g per serving. For that reason, the ingredients list is still probably your best source of information.

The maximum amount of trans fats you should allow in your diet per day is less than 1 percent of total calories, which comes to 1.8 g on an 1,800-calorie diet. That means, for the most part, you'll need to avoid just about all foods that contain partially hydrogenated vegetable oils. Occasionally, I will recommend foods that contain some partially hydrogenated oil, but in levels so low that the trans fat content is listed as zero on the nutrition panel; you can safely work them into your diet on days when your diet has been free and

OTHER HEALTHY OILS

Although olive oil and canola oil should be the staples of any healthy kitchen, there are also several other types of nutritious oils on store shelves that you can use to supplement olive and canola. Most of them also have a fairly pungent and interesting flavor, so you don't need to use a lot to add some punch to food. The following are ones to look for:

Toasted sesame oil: Rich in vitamin E, it has a fairly strong flavor and is best in Asian dressings and dishes.

Walnut oil: This type of oil may lower triglycerides and is best in salads.

Peanut oil: Contains a phytochemical called resveratrol that lowers the risk of heart disease and cancer, and you can use this as you would use canola oil, including in cooking.

Grapeseed oil: Virtually flavorless, it may reduce LDL cholesterol.

clear of other sources of trans fats. And the very few that I do recommend have other compelling benefits such as fiber and vitamins and minerals.

What to Have Instead: Healthy Fats When it comes to fats, olive oil, which is rich in cholesterol-lowering monounsaturated fat, is my top pick. You're probably not going to find too many baked goods or processed products made with olive oil (though there are some), so look for those made with other healthy oils such as canola, high-oleic safflower, or high-oleic sunflower oil. For your own home use, though, I recommend olive oil or, if you prefer, the blander-tasting canola oil.

Oils that are cold-pressed aren't exposed to as much heat as regular oils and do not form trans fat. Extra-virgin and virgin olive oils are cold-pressed, and always the best choice. If you can find and afford them, give cold-pressed oils a try; they are generally more flavorful and contain healthful phytonutrients.

I still meet many people trying to lose weight who are afraid of using any oil at all. There was some validity to the low- (or no-) fat craze that took hold several years ago; however, the pendulum swung too far. Healthy fats are an essential part of your diet not only because they provide important nutrients like vitamin E and omega-3 fatty acids, but also because they add tremendous flavor to food and make eating more enjoyable. And because fat helps slow digestion, it helps you stay fuller longer, too.

However, you still have to be careful about including fat in your diet. At 9 calories per gram, fat has more calories than protein or carbohydrates, which only have 4 each. I recommend that your fat intake be 25 to 35 percent of your total calories, a ratio that you'll find built into the meals on the Best Life Diet Meal Plans. Taking fried food off your menu, scaling back to nonfat or low-fat dairy, reducing the amount of oil in your salad dressings, and topping baked potatoes with salsa instead of sour cream are ways to keep your fat intake in check. And, as I've been saying, not all fats are created equal. Keep the saturated fat you get from animal foods like meat and cheese to a minimum and stick with olive and canola oil, supplementing them with some of the other healthy oils I mention on page 104.

If you're going to use butter, which contains saturated fat, use it only occasionally and sparingly. Whenever possible, substitute olive or canola oil for the butter called for in recipes. These days, I even use a mild-tasting olive oil to cook eggs. If you don't particularly like the taste of olive oil, try the light versions (but be forewarned that in this case "light" refers to the color and flavor, *not* the calories). If you must have some kind of butter-like spread on your toast, look for one of the margarine spreads with labels stating "0 g trans fat" (some margarines still contain trans fats). You may also consider switching to peanut butter or another nut spread. I'll talk more about those in Phase Three.

FRIED FOODS

I've been sitting back, listening to what I think is a sort of ironic debate about fried foods. There's been a big outcry about the fact that many restaurants deep-fry their foods in trans fats. Hands have been wrung and lawsuits have been filed, all in the name of getting the trans fats out of fried food.

Obviously, I'm no fan of trans fats—I've just told you to eliminate them from your diet. And if you're going to have fried foods once in a while as a treat, I'd of course want them to be free of trans fats (and at this point, despite the uproar, most fried foods still *do* contain trans fats). But the real outcry shouldn't be only about what's being used to fry food, but also about the fact that fried food is eaten in excess by many Americans. If there is a campaign that's worth waging, that's it. Fried food doesn't belong in a healthful diet except on the rarest of occasions.

Even if there is not a trace of trans fat in a serving of fried chicken, fried fish, French fries, or onion rings, fried food made in restaurants is often cooked in oil that's used over and over again. This can cause the development of by-products that have been linked to a variety of diseases, including cancer.

And no matter what type of oil fried food is cooked in, it's highly caloric. A recent Harvard study found that the more fried food adolescents ate, the more they weighed, and I wouldn't be surprised if the same was true of adults. Particularly now, in Phase Two, when significant weight loss is your goal, fried food is off-limits.

What to Have Instead: Oven-Fried Foods If you feel that you can't give up potato chips, at least look for baked varieties made without trans fats (baked chips still contain oil, just not as much of it as fried chips). And at home, try oven-fried foods as a substitute. To make oven-fried "fries," cut potatoes into strips, toss them with a little olive oil (or spritz them lightly with an olive oil spray), season with salt and pepper, and cook them in a 400-degree oven until toasty brown. Even better, use peeled sweet potatoes or carrots, which are rich in the antioxidant beta-carotene.

If you love fried chicken, you may also go for the oven-fried version: dip skinless chicken breasts in beaten egg (or a mix of lemon juice and water), then roll them in seasoned bread crumbs or crushed cornflakes that have been spiked with your favorite seasonings. Bake until the chicken is cooked through.

WHITE BREAD

Unlike many diet programs, the Best Life Diet doesn't prohibit you from eating carbohydrates. What it does, though, is get you to switch over to whole grain carbs a little at a time, starting with the elimination of white bread. White bread is made from refined grains, and refined grains are stripped of their germ and outer bran layer, and therefore most of their nutritional value. Taking away the bran and germ makes grains smooth and palatable (think of how easy white bread goes down), but it also re-

GREAT WHOLE GRAIN PICKS

Here are some whole grain breads and pastas I like. Still, check the ingredient list of each product, since formulations can change.

100 PERCENT WHOLE GRAIN BREADS

Country Hearth 100 percent whole wheat bread

Arnold Bakery Light 100 percent whole wheat bread

Thomas's Sahara whole wheat pita

Flatout multigrain wraps

Pepperidge Farm whole grain breads

Rudi's Organic Bakery wheat and oat bread

Thomas' Hearty Grains 100 percent whole wheat English muffins and 100 percent whole wheat bagels

Pepperidge Farm 100 percent whole wheat English muffins and 100 percent whole wheat bagels

Wasa crispbread (kind of a cross between bread and a cracker), whole grain varieties

PASTAS THAT ARE WHOLE GRAIN OR HAVE ADDED FIBER

Barilla PLUS

Barilla Whole Grain

Bionaturae whole durum wheat

Eden Foods spelt whole grain

moves most of their fiber, B vitamins, vitamin E, and disease-fighting phytochemicals. Whole grains, however, come with the bran and germ. That may be why they are also associated with a wide range of health benefits that refined grains are not, including helping to promote a reduced risk of heart disease; stomach, colon, and ovarian cancers; and diabetes. Then there's the fiber. Breads made with 100 percent whole wheat or other whole grains have two to three times the fiber of white bread. As I discussed earlier in the section on hunger, high-fiber foods are bulkier and processed more slowly by the body than other types of foods, which helps keep you fuller longer. When people add fiber to their diets, they eat fewer calories and shed pounds.

In the original edition of this book, I also asked readers to eliminate regular pasta and eat only fiber-enriched or 100 percent whole grain pastas. I wanted you to get the phytonutrients and increased fiber (four times as much) that these pastas have over regula pasta. I'm dropping that requirement in this edition for two reasons. The first is that even regular pasta is a healthful food. As I explained in the original edition, regular pasta is made with a type of wheat flour called semolina—cracked wheat—which does have some benefits, even when it's not in a whole grain form. The wheat particles in semolina are much bigger than the pulverized flour particles found in most refined flours. Their size makes it difficult for your body to convert regular pasta to blood sugar quickly, so pasta doesn't send your blood sugar level soaring (and then crashing down) the way other foods made from refined flours can. That means it will help keep you satisfied for a fairly long time, always a plus when you're trying to lose weight. The other reason I've put it back on the table is because it's still so hard to find whole grain pasta in restaurants and in frozen and take-out foods. I don't want to prevent you from having an otherwise nutritious meal just because it contains regular pasta. For instance, the healthiest item at an Italian restaurant might be regular pasta topped with marinara sauce and grilled chicken (always avoid the creamy sauces).

I'd still recommend that you make the switch to whole grain or fiber-enriched pasta (like Barilla PLUS) whenever you're cooking at home. But I recognize that many people just don't like the taste and texture of 100 percent whole grain pasta. Fortunately, there are high-fiber pastas out there that taste similar to regular pasta—check the label for at least 4 g of fiber per 2 ounces of dried pasta. Two that have the Best Life seal on them are Barilla PLUS and Barilla Whole Grain.

I happen to love regular pasta, and I use my own Anything Goes calories to have it once in a while. (I stick to a reasonably sized portion—one to two cups—just like the Italians do.) You can still keep some of the familiar refined grains such as white rice and crackers made with refined flour in your diet for now if you really want to, but later, in Phase Three, you're going to move even closer to an almost all whole grain foods diet.

What to Eat Instead: Whole Grain Bread When low-carbohydrate, high-protein diets became popular a few years ago, sales of bread, pasta, rice, and other grain foods slumped. Thankfully, these carbs, which are a good source of energy, particularly for active people who need carbohydrates to fuel their muscles, are back in favor. Better yet, you can now find more whole grain versions of them than ever before, including some really great whole grain breads.

If you don't often (or ever) eat whole grain carbs, it may take you a while to get used to them: they tend to be chewier and more intensely flavored. The good news is that many food manufacturers are working on making whole grain foods a little lighter in texture and taste, and there are already a few improved products on the market.

One thing you should be aware of, though, is that it's not always easy to tell if a grain food—and not just bread and pasta, but crackers, cereals, and frozen waffles, among other processed foods—contains a meaningful amount of whole grains. Some "wheat" breads don't contain any whole wheat (or very little of it) even though they're brown in color. And now that whole grains are on more health-conscious people's radar, some manufacturers are putting words like *whole grain* and *multigrain* on food labels even though their products don't contain much whole grain at all.

Always check ingredient lists; that's where the truth lies. The ingredients that make up the largest percentage of a food are always listed first, so you want to make sure that whole grains are at the top of the list (and if it's wheat, make sure it has the word *whole* in front of it, as in "whole wheat flour"). A product doesn't have to be made entirely of whole grains to be nutritious, but the whole grains should be the prime ingredients. You can also check the nutrition panel to see what the food's fiber content is: there's no set amount of fiber that indicates whole grains were used to make a product. However, if a bread has at least 2 g of fiber per slice, it has some whole grain or added fiber (also a good thing)

The Whole Grains Council issues Whole Grain Stamps, seals that food manufacturers can put on their products to alert shoppers to their whole grain content. To receive a stamp, a product must have at least 8 g of whole grain per serving. Stamps marked "100%" mean that all the grain in that product is whole, and it contains at least 16 g of whole grain per serving. (The USDA and other health institutions consider 16 g a grain serving.) Look for these golden stamps as you make your way down super-market aisles.

HIGH-FAT MILK AND YOGURT

Dairy products, as you probably already know, are excellent sources of calcium and protein, so it's a good idea to keep them in your diet. However, especially when it comes to milk and yogurt, there's absolutely no reason to have full-fat versions; even 2 percent products have more fat than you need. The fat in dairy products is saturated, the kind that is linked with clogged arteries, and whole milk dairy products contain about five times as much cholesterol as nonfat. And, of course, whole milk and 2 percent dairy products are much higher in calories than their nonfat counterparts.

What to Eat Instead: Nonfat or 1 Percent Dairy Products If you still consume whole milk or 2 percent dairy products, switch to skim or at least 1 percent. The nutrition stats make the difference plain:

> **1 CUP WHOLE MILK:** 146 calories, 7.9 g fat, 4.5 g saturated fat, 24 mg cholesterol

> **1 CUP 2 PERCENT MILK:** 122 calories, 4.8 g fat, 3.1 g saturated fat, 20 mg cholesterol

> **1 CUP 1 PERCENT MILK:** 103 calories, 2.3 g fat, 1.5 g saturated fat, 12 mg cholesterol

> **1 CUP NONFAT MILK:** 83 calories, 0.2 g fat, 0.2 g saturated fat, 5 mg cholesterol

Besides a substantial nutritional difference, there's a substantial flavor (and texture) difference between whole and both 1 percent and nonfat milk and yogurt. It's for that reason that most people generally have a hard time with the lower-fat milk products at first, but after a while, their taste buds adapt and they actually prefer them; whole milk eventually tastes too rich. I've worked my way down to using nonfat milk in my smoothies, but I haven't been able to quite make the complete leap—I still use 1 percent milk in my cereal. It's one of the concessions that I can afford to make because I exercise so much. But for weight-loss purposes, I still think that nonfat is the way to go. So see if you can get all the way down to nonfat. If it's just too watery for you, settle for 1 percent.

While an ounce of regular (whole fat) cheese daily is okay, that's not quite enough to make a cheese sandwich. So if cheese is a staple, make the switch to reduced fat (about 5 g fat per ounce). Cabot 50% Reduced Fat Cheddar is one of my favorites. Skip nonfat cheese—it's awful-tasting.

Judging Your Success

The main goals of Phase Two are to help you understand and gauge your hunger, get your portions down to size, toss out some foods that either contain too many empty calories or too much fat, and in doing so, consistently drop a significant number of pounds. A sign that you've made the changeover successfully is that you are losing steadily at a rate of about 1 to 2 pounds a week. At the end of four weeks, though, you have to make a decision about what to do next. Here are some guidelines to help you.

IF YOU'VE MET YOUR GOAL WEIGHT
This is the best of all possible worlds. Move on to Phase Three, where you can continue making dietary changes that will help you maintain the weight loss, improve your health, and give you a road map to a lifetime of nutritious eating.

IF YOU ARE 20 POUNDS OR LESS FROM YOUR GOAL WEIGHT AND ARE STILL CONSISTENTLY DROPPING POUNDS
You have a couple of options. You can stay in Phase Two until you reach your goal or you stop losing, then move on to Phase Three, or you can move on to Phase Three right now. In Phase Three, your weight loss may be slightly slower; however, you can begin taking immediate advantage of new dietary changes that are going to benefit your health greatly.

IF YOU STILL HAVE MORE THAN 20 POUNDS TO LOSE AND ARE STILL CONSISTENTLY DROPPING POUNDS
Just keep doing what you're doing. Stay in Phase Two—it's working!

IF YOU ARE 20 POUNDS OR MORE FROM YOUR GOAL WEIGHT AND HAVE STOPPED DROPPING POUNDS

I want you to make sure that you are fulfilling all of the Phase One and the Phase Two objectives and that you haven't unconsciously let extra calories slip back into you diet (keeping a food diary for a week can help you get a good picture of what's really going on). Have you been inconsistent or maybe even cheated a bit? If you find you've strayed, recommit to and re-instate all the Phase One and Phase Two changes. If you haven't strayed, either cut your calories a little more or increase your exercise or both. It's possible that you have hit a plateau, and one or both of these changes will get your weight loss moving again. If you continue to have trouble losing, there are a couple of things I want you to think about.

The first is whether or not your weight-loss goal is realistic in the first place. Take your genetics, your body type, and your lifestyle into account and assess how much you can reasonably lose. It may be that you really can't go any further than you have without significantly disrupting your life with too much exercise and too little food.

The other thing I want you to think about is how badly you want to drop those last pounds. Is it so important that you are willing to sacrifice some of the things that give you pleasure in your life—like time with friends and family, restaurant meals, and absolutely all of your favorite foods—to achieve your goal? It's a question Oprah eventually had to ask herself. For a long time, she was stuck on getting her weight down to a par-ticular number, but at some point, she realized it would mean devoting so much time to working out and eating so restrictively that she would have much less joy in her life. That's absolutely contrary to what this program stands for. It's about having your best *life*. Trying to lose weight beyond a point where your body is vigorously fighting it can keep you from really liv-ing your life. You've got to ask yourself if it's worth the effort; maybe it is or maybe it's not.

If you decide that it's not, move on to Phase Three. Instituting all the changes in that phase is going to allow you to take control of your health and well-being without putting a lot of strain on your life.

PHASE THREE

▶ When you arrive at Phase Three, you'll have come far down the road toward establishing good eating practices. Now you're going to continue to upgrade your diet by tossing out more of the empty calories and replacing them with wholesome, nutritious foods. If you still have weight to lose during this phase, you'll find some tips to help you do so on page 118. But whether you're going to continue to lose or are already at your goal weight, I want to begin shifting your focus to improving the quality of your diet.

Starting now, your main goal should be to fill your day with the healthiest food you can find, using all the recipes and food recommendations throughout this book, the information on my website, and healthy, high-quality products such as those with the Best Life seal of approval on them to help you. And when I say high quality, I don't mean expensive. What I mean is food that has a natural goodness (like a perfectly ripe peach or plate of barbecued shrimp and grilled vegetables), is free of unhealthy ingredients, and is going to help you lock in the weight loss you achieved in Phases One and Two. Just about every food you eat should offer you great taste, vitamins, minerals, and the other nutrients you need for both satisfaction and good health. That's my definition of a high-quality food.

On the following pages, I'm going to map it all out for you and present you with the guidelines to live by. Within those guidelines, I'm also going to introduce you to the concept of Anything Goes calories. These are calories that you can use to incorporate foods into your diet that aren't necessarily the most healthful choices, but when eaten in moderation, won't impact your health or weight and will keep you from feeling deprived. Anything Goes calories don't have to be spent on junk. It's a better idea, I think, to put them toward treats that, while indulgent, also have redeeming qualities, such as healthy fats or disease-fighting phytonutrients. A glass of wine, a chunk of dark chocolate, a dish of fruit crisp are the ideal kinds of Anything Goes food, but the calories are yours, and you're free to use them as you please. (See page 120 for more healthy Anything Goes treats.)

Phase Three is, in fact, about grabbing the reins and deciding how you want to eat for the rest of your life. You may find that the changes I suggest are right on target and that you're comfortable following them to the letter. You may decide that you want a diet that is slightly more forgiving, with more leeway to eat foods that I recommend eliminating. Or you may choose to go even further by ridding your diet of anything nutritionally substandard and devoting your Anything Goes calories solely toward 100 percent healthy foods. It's all within *your* control.

PHASE THREE

TIME FRAME: The rest of your life

WEIGH IN: Continue to weigh in no more than once a week, no less than once a month

FOCUS: Improving the quality of your diet for good health and lifelong weight maintenance

OBJECTIVES:

▶ Build on the changes you made in Phases One and Two:

   ▷ Live an active life

   ▷ Eat three meals, including a nutritious breakfast, plus at least one snack daily

   ▷ Stop eating at least two hours before bedtime

   ▷ Stay hydrated

   ▷ Bolster your diet with daily supplements

   ▷ Understand the physical nature of your hunger

   ▷ Understand the emotional reasons for your hunger

   ▷ Use the hunger scale

   ▷ Eat reasonable portions

   ▷ Remove six unhealthy foods from your diet

▶ Increase your activity at least one level (optional)

▶ Introduce Anything Goes calories into your regimen

▶ Balance your diet using the Best Life Diet Guidelines

▶ Remove more unhealthy foods from your diet

▶ Add more wholesome foods to your diet

JUDGING YOUR SUCCESS: Decide how you want to live your best life and live it

I don't expect you to incorporate all the recommendations in Phase Three into your diet at once; do the best you can and keep working toward maintaining the best possible diet. Consider the way you eat a work in progress. My own diet is quite good, but I'm still always looking for ways to improve it. I know that I eat better now than I did in years past, and I hope to eat even more healthfully in the years to come. The way you eat, like everything else in life, should evolve, and I hope you'll use the www.thebestlife.com website to help you keep the process going.

TIME FRAME

This is your diet for life.

WEIGH IN

If you're still trying to lose some weight, then follow the weigh-in guidelines for Phase Two and weigh yourself weekly. But if you don't need to lose more weight, then how you handle the scale is a personal choice. Some of you will do best with a monthly check to make sure that you're where you want to be, but if you gain weight easily, regular weekly weigh-ins may still be a good idea. This way you nip small weight gains in the bud, before they get bigger. That said, you don't want to become preoccupied with the scale or let it make you crazy (remember, there are lots of reasons why body weight fluctuates naturally); in general, you should weigh yourself no more than once a week and no less than once a month. If you have a tendency to take the numbers a little too seriously, use a favorite pair of pants to keep you posted on how you're doing. If the waist feels a little too tight, you'll know it's time to cut back a bit.

PHASE THREE OBJECTIVES

Build on the Changes You Made in Phase One and Phase Two

During Phase Three, you have the choice of continuing to lose weight or maintaining your weight. There is a subtle difference between the two, and the key is your use of the hunger scale. If you want to continue to achieve a calorie deficit to shed those last few pounds, use the rule you used in Phase Two to determine when you should cease eating: put your fork down when you hit a 5 on the hunger scale. Stopping at 5 is going to ensure that you don't eat more calories than you burn. Also, continue to pause before deciding if you should go for seconds or have dessert (or even if you should finish everything on your plate). Giving the appetite mechanisms that signal your brain to put the brakes on time to do their job is going to have a significant impact on how hungry you feel and, subsequently, your daily calorie intake. If you're working to maintain your weight loss, you can now move your stopping point up a notch to level 6 on the hunger scale. This will allow you to eat slightly more food, but not so much that the pounds will reappear.

Besides continuing to use the hunger scale to control your appetite, you're also going to maintain all the changes you made in Phases One and Two, perhaps with the exception of eliminating alcohol.

Increase Your Activity at Least One Level (Optional)

Just as you are now about to make refining your diet an ongoing project, it will be to your benefit to make refining your activity a continuing goal. One of the great things about activity is that any and all exercise you do trains your body to be ready for an even greater challenge. The hardest part is getting started; after that, your body adapts, and it gets easier and easier to increase how much you move.

I want you to be realistic about how much activity your life will allow, but I also want to urge you to be creative. Maybe you can't start, or have no interest in starting, the formal aerobic workouts in activity level 2, but you can add twenty minutes of strength-training twice a week to your regimen. If you don't like strength-training, maybe you can go to a calisthenics, yoga, or circuit weight-training class twice a week.

The guidelines of the Best Life Activity Scale (page 44) are just that: guidelines. I encourage you to think outside the box if it will help you include more activity into your life. Increasing your activity is not only going to help you maintain the weight loss you've achieved and allow you to eat more food without regaining weight (take note: the higher your activity level, the more Anything Goes calories you'll be rewarded with), but it's also going to help slow down the aging process. That's just one more reason you should make exercise an ongoing part of your life.

Introduce Anything Goes Calories into Your Regimen

I've been teasing you with the idea of using Anything Goes calories throughout this book, and now you're finally going to get to use them! Let me explain in greater detail what they are and why they enter into your diet at Phase Three.

You get a certain number of Anything Goes calories each day; how many depends on how much activity you do. (If, however, you're a woman at Level 0, you don't get any Anything Goes calories, a good reason to move up to at least activity level 1.) If you're trying to adhere to the calorie recommendations in the Best Life Diet Guidelines (page 125), bear in mind that those recommendations take your Anything Goes calories into consideration. If you're at calorie level 1,800, that number already includes the 210 calories you may use in any way you see fit.

Anything Goes calories give you a chance to eat foods that, despite cleaning up most of your diet, you still have a hankering for; that is, they give you a chance to eat foods that, truthfully, don't have all that much to recommend them. They may be foods with very, very empty calories, such as candy bars, cookies, or potato chips. They may be foods that contain ingredients like saturated fat or sodium that you'd never want to eat in large quantities. Some examples include French fries, doughnuts, and nondairy creamer, all of which also generally contain trans fats; the kind of microwave popcorn that's high in fat and contains a boatload of salt; heavily marbled steaks or butter on your bread, which are sources of saturated fat;

candy bars and oversized, super-sweet muffins, which are full of sugar (and sometimes too much fat) and not much else. As I mentioned earlier, my preference is that you put your Anything Goes calories toward "luxury foods" that are indulgent, but still have something beneficial to offer, such as dark chocolate, chocolate milk, or whole milk yogurt (high in saturated fat, but all good sources of calcium); reduced-fat, 0 grams trans fat popcorn (a good source of fiber); a berry sorbet or fruit crumble (high in sugar but a source of antioxidants); or a glass of wine (which contains disease-fighting phytonutrients).

To make it easy to spot high-quality Anything Goes options, I've given select products the Best Life Treat seal. Sweets and snacks carrying this seal contain no more than 150 calories, are free of partially hydrogenated oil, and have other health perks. (A list of products with this seal can be found on my website, www.thebestlife.com.)

Anything Goes calories are still a relatively small percentage of your total daily calories. They're just enough to allow you to treat yourself, but not enough to junk up your overall diet or send your calorie count over the top. You still have to watch your portion sizes: for instance, if you decide to have an oversized muffin but have just 150 Anything Goes calories, you'll probably have to limit yourself to just half or a quarter of the muffin. Or if you want to have the occasional splurge on something that is very high in calories, like a big fat-marbled steak or tall ice cream sundae,

ANYTHING GOES CALORIES

Activity Level	Women	Men
0	0	100
1	100	150
2	150	210
3	210	280
4	280	300
5	300	350

then you may have to skip your Anything Goes calories for a few days to have enough for an oversized treat.

In the following sections, I'll give you more details about what foods should be considered Anything Goes calories. Check out the table above to determine your daily ration.

A NOTE ON THE FOODS YOU ELIMINATED IN PHASE TWO

All of the foods you pulled out of your diet in Phase Two should be considered Anything Goes calories: soda; foods that contain trans fats—even ones like some crackers and ramen soups; all fried foods, from onion rings to potato chips to fried chicken and fried fish; white bread, even baguettes and sourdough loaves; and most high-fat dairy foods such as ice cream and whipped cream. High-fat cheeses, because they're a good source of calcium and protein and don't contain sugar, can fit into your regular diet as long as you use them sparingly (about one ounce daily). A latte made with nonfat or 1 percent milk isn't Anything Goes, but a latte made with 2 percent or whole milk (much higher in saturated fat) is—as is a frozen blended drink, which is filled with sugar. Some low-fat dairy products, because of the double whammy of fat and sugar, should also be considered Anything Goes calories, including flavored milks, milkshakes, and frozen yogurt.

Preferred Anything Goes Choices

Wine: May have heart-protective benefits.

Dark chocolate: Contains disease-fighting phytonutrients (which milk chocolate does not).

Fruit juice: A good source of vitamins and, if it contains pulp, some fiber. Your first four ounces of juice for the day doesn't have to be an Anything Goes beverage; however, if you're going to have more, the rest should be.

Fruit desserts: Like juice, a good source of vitamins and some fiber.

Sweetened iced tea: Black tea may help protect against heart disease and stroke; green and black teas may boost the immune system.

White-flour pretzels: Although they don't really bring nutrients to the table, they are moderate in calories and provide a satisfying crunch.

White-flour baguette: Ditto (minus the crunch).

Full-fat cheese: A good source of calcium.

Full-fat yogurt: Ditto.

Flavored low-fat or nonfat milk: Ditto again.

Pizza: Despite the fat from the cheese, this food offers lycopene (from the tomato sauce) and calcium (from the cheese). But if you have pizza with low-fat cheese and whole grain crust, it can be part of your regular, not Anything Goes, Best Life plan.

Whole wheat graham crackers: While these are pretty sweet, they also contain fiber.

Granola bars: The better ones have no more than 12 g sugar and at least 2 g fiber and about 150 to 180 calories.

Oatmeal cookies: They'll contribute a little fiber and whole grain to your diet.

Balance Your Diet Using the Best Life Diet Guidelines

All foods are not created equal; you need more of some than others. The Best Life Diet Guidelines, outlined in the chart on page 125, sum up how you should be dividing your diet to ensure that you consume all the nutrients you need without going over your calorie limits or eating too much of the foods that you *don't* need. More specifically, the foods that you don't need (or, in the case of sodium, don't need much of) are saturated fats, trans fats, added sugar, and sodium. A healthful diet can incorporate just about anything within reason, but you especially have to take "within reason" to heart when it comes to foods that can adversely affect your health.

The Best Life Diet Guidelines provide you with both the number of servings of healthy foods you need each day and the maximum amounts of saturated fat, trans fats, added sugar, and sodium your diet should include. When you look at the chart, what you'll see essentially is a blueprint of what a nutritious diet should look like: rich in fruits, vegetables, whole grains, and sources of lean protein; moderate in dairy and healthy fats; and low in unhealthy fats, sugar, and sodium.

MINIMIZE YOUR INTAKE:
FOUR TO WATCH OUT FOR

Saturated Fat

The primary source of saturated fat, known to raise LDL ("bad") cholesterol levels and increase the risk of heart disease, is animal foods like fatty
meats, whole and 2 percent dairy, and poultry skin. Some health organizations recommend limiting saturated fat to 7 percent of total calories
daily, others to just under 10 percent. If you can get down to 7 percent, I
think it's a good idea. If not, 9 percent is a happy medium, and that's the
percentage I've used to calculate the allowances in the Best Life Diet
Guidelines.

Whittling your way down to nonfat or 1 percent dairy in Phase Two
and then switching to lean-protein sources in Phase Three should allow
you to easily stay within a healthful range. However, always check the nutrition information on all packaged foods you eat—saturated fat, which is
also present in palm oil, palm kernel oil, coconut milk, and coconut oil, is
often lurking where you least expect it. (Some research suggests that the
type of saturated fat in coconut oil may not be as harmful as that in other
sources, but scientists are still sorting this out. Until they do, better to err
on the side of caution.) Food manufacturers are required to list saturated-
fat content on the package, which helps you be a conscientious shopper.

Trans Fats

In Phase Two, you began your mission to remove as many sources of trans
fats from your diet as possible (see page 102 for the full rundown). Your
ultimate goal should be to get your intake of these artery-clogging fats as
close to zero as possible. Look for partially hydrogenated oils on the ingredients list—that's your clue that trans fats are hiding inside.

Added Sugar

Most high-sugar foods are just empty calories. Added sugar doesn't only refer to the sugar you spoon into your coffee; it also includes the sugars that are found in baked goods, cereals, sweetened drinks, and other processed foods. Sugar is listed on the nutrition facts panel of most products, which helps you get your daily tally, though the nutrition facts panel lumps together both naturally occurring and added sugar. For instance, a raisin bran cereal contains both naturally occurring sugar from the raisins and some sugar added to the cereal itself, but the food label won't tell you which is which (consumer watchdog groups are lobbying the Food and Drug Administration [FDA] to change this). So the best you can do is look at the ingredient list; if sugar, high-fructose corn syrup, fruit juice sweetener, honey, fructose, dextrose, maltose, or any other sweeteners are among the first three ingredients, it's likely that much of the sugar is added.

Sodium

Even if you rarely use the salt shaker yourself, you may be getting much more sodium than you're aware of. It's used—liberally—in almost all packaged foods. Sodium is associated with high blood pressure, though some people seem to be more prone to its effects than others. Since salt is a preservative as well as a flavor enhancer, many manufacturers use a heavy hand with the salt shaker. In general, try to keep your sodium intake below 350 mg at breakfast; under 600 mg at lunch; under 650 mg at dinner; and under 300 mg for snacks, which also helps you keep your daily intake to recommended levels. Relegate high-sodium snacks that don't seem so bad, such as pretzels (unless they're whole grain and unsalted) and baked chips, to the Anything Goes category.

THE BEST LIFE DIET GUIDELINES

To map out your own personal Best Life diet, you simply need to know your activity level. I've done all of the calculations for you. Here's how to put together a balanced diet and estimate a daily calorie level.

1 *Find your activity level.* If you need a refresher, go to page 46 and see where you fall on the 0–5 Best Life Activity Scale.

2 *Find your calorie level.* Next to your activity level on the first chart on the opposite page, you'll see a corresponding calorie level. This is an estimate of the number of calories you'll need per day based on how much you move. Obviously, I can't know everything about you that may affect how many calories you actually burn, so consider these calorie levels somewhat flexible. If you're not losing enough weight or if you're having a hard time sticking to a calorie level, go up or down accordingly (just don't drop below 1,200 calories, because it's difficult to get enough of the nutrients that you need on a diet any more restrictive than that). For instance, if you are a woman at activity Level 2 and not losing weight while consuming 1,700 calories per day, then drop down to 1,600. If you're losing weight but are constantly too hungry while consuming 1,700 calories per day, go up to 1,800. I'd rather have you lose weight at a slower pace than jump ship because you feel deprived.

   Remember that your Anything Goes calories are already figured into your daily calorie count—they're not calories over and above your daily total.

3 *Find your serving allowances.* Check out the Number of Servings per Daily Activity Level chart on the opposite page. The letters (A, B, C, D, E, and F) correspond to calorie levels in the chart above. Notice that servings of healthful foods *and* Anything Goes calories are included in each calorie level. For example, if you're a B, the healthy foods come to 1,500 calories and the Anything Goes calories make up the final 100 calories, to tally 1,600 calories.

Daily Calories per Activity Level

Women Activity Level 0 (1,500 cals.)	A
Women Activity Level 1/Men Activity Level 0 (1,600 cals.)	B
Women Activity Level 2/Men Activity Level 1 (1,700 cals.)	C
Women Activity Level 3/Men Activity Level 2 (1,800 cals.)	D
Women Activity Levels 4 and 5*/Men Activity Levels 3 and 4 (2,000 cals.)	E
Women Activity Level 5* (2,500 cals.)/Men Activity Level 5 (2,500–2,550 cals.)	F

*At Activity Level 5 some women need around 2,000 calories; others can go up to 2,500.

Nutritious Foods	Number of Servings per Daily Activity Level					
	A	B	C	D	E	F
Grains/starchy vegetables*	5	5	5	$5^1/_2$	6	9
Fruit	2	2	2	2	2	3
Vegetables	4	4	5	6	6	7
Dairy (nonfat or 1%)	2	2	2	2	2	3
Protein-rich foods	6	7	7	7	7	8
Healthy fat	5	5	5	5	7	7
Anything Goes cals., women	0	100	150	210	280	300
Anything Goes cals., men	0	100	150	210	280	350

*Starchy vegetables include potatoes, corn, and peas.

Food Components to Limit	Maximum Amounts					
Saturated fat (less than 10% of total calories)	15 g	16 g	17 g	18 g	20 g	25 g
Trans fats (less than 1% of total calories)	1.5 g	1.6 g	1.7 g	1.8 g	2 g	2.5 g
Added sugar	37 g	40 g	43 g	45 g	50 g	64 g
Sodium	2,300 mg (all levels)					

4 *Get familiar with serving sizes.* Use the What's a Serving? chart on page 126 to gauge reasonable portions of oatmeal, rice, steak, fish, salad dressing, and other foods.

5 *Find your maximums for the four food components you should limit.* Check out the Food Components to Limit above. Remember that these are the maximum numbers for saturated fat, trans fat, sugar, and sodium. If possible, keep your intake of these four even lower.

What's a Serving?

Food Group	A Serving Is About . . .	A Serving Looks Like . . .
Grains (preferably whole grains) or starchy vegetables	80 calories	1/2 cup of brown rice, whole wheat or fiber-enriched pasta, or hot whole grain cereal; about 1 cup of cold whole grain cereal; 1 slice of whole grain bread; one 6-inch tortilla; 1/4 large bagel; 1/2 medium bagel or English muffin; 1/2 cup potato, sweet potato, or corn
Fruit	60 calories	1 medium-size fruit or 1 cup of chopped fruit or berries; 1/2 cup of grapes; 2 tablespoons of dried fruit; 1/2 cup of fruit juice
Vegetables	25 calories	1–2 cups of raw leafy vegetables; 1/2 cup of chopped nonleafy vegetables; 1/2 cup of cooked vegetables; 3/4 cup of tomato juice
Dairy	100 calories	1 cup of nonfat or 1% milk or 3/4 cup of plain low-fat or nonfat yogurt; 1 cup of calcium-enriched soymilk (no more than 100 calories per cup); 1 1/2 ounces reduced-fat hard or semi-hard cheese; or 1 ounce regular cheese*
Protein	65 calories	1 ounce of lean meat, poultry, or fish; 1/3 cup of tofu or tempeh; 1/3 cup of cooked beans; 1 egg; 1/3 cup of 1% or 2% cottage cheese; 1 1/2 ounce of reduced-fat hard or semi-hard cheese; 1 ounce regular cheese*; 1 tablespoon of peanut butter*
Healthy fats	45 calories	1 teaspoon of olive or canola oil; 1 tablespoon of olive or canola oil-based salad dressing; 3 tablespoons of chopped avocado; 1 tablespoon of almonds, pecans, cashews, peanuts, or walnuts; 1 tablespoon of ground flaxseed; 1 1/2 teaspoons of peanut or almond butter or tahini; 8 olives

* If you have this higher-fat choice, then you have used up one of your fat servings, too.

How Many Servings per Meal?

To fulfill the Best Life Diet Guidelines, you'll need to know what exactly constitutes a serving; this is important because most people tend to overestimate serving sizes. In fact, in some cases you may be surprised at how small servings of certain foods seem (for example, a quarter of a large bagel is equal to one serving), but keep in mind that you don't have to have just one serving at a sitting. Your morning bowl of oatmeal or cold cereal can be two servings, as you'll see in our meal plans. And a salad can have two to three servings of vegetables or, depending on the type of salad, even more. In fact, a salad is a great way to cover most of your vegetable requirement for the day in one shot. The point is to meet your daily requirements. That—and using the hunger scale—will ensure that you don't overeat.

Remove More Unhealthy Foods from Your Diet

If I had asked you in the first phase of this program to give up high-fat sources of protein like hamburgers, sweets like cookies and candy, and greasy snacks like potato chips, you probably could have done so without any problem—*for a while*. But how long would you have been able to resist them? Now that you've adopted some other healthy behaviors—you're active, consuming regular meals and snacks, using the hunger scale, and making changes to eliminate emotional eating—you have habits in place that are going to make you feel less compelled to eat junky foods. So when you do eliminate most of them from your diet, the chances are greater that your decision is going to stick.

One reason why fatty, sugary, and salty foods are so prominent in the American diet is convenience. What's easier than pulling a chocolate bar from a vending machine or whizzing by a fast-food drive-thru for a soda burger, and fries? At least that's the way most people think. But it's a myth that only unhealthy foods are convenient. Many fast-food restaurants and convenience stores also have healthful choices; it's just as easy to grab a banana at the 7-Eleven or the Asian salad with grilled chicken or the Fruit 'n Yogurt Parfait at McDonald's.

That's one option. Another one: Be prepared. If you're like most people, you probably follow a fairly regular routine, or, at the very least, you know where you're going to be and what you're going to be doing most of the day. So plan for it. If you know that you're going to be sitting at your desk at 3 P.M., struggling to keep your eyes open because you need a snack, have one of the snacks on page 59 in your desk drawer or in the office refrigerator. If you know you're going to be in your car shuttling your kids around all day, don't leave yourself at the mercy of unhealthy quick-energy solutions: pack a lunch and/or some healthful snacks so that you don't find yourself at the drive-thru ordering French fries. If you're dining out, choose places where you know they have dishes that meet the Best Life Diet criteria and don't let anyone bully you into deviating from the healthful way you want to eat. Good food is out there; you just need to make sure that it's always available to you.

HIGH-FAT MEATS

Since it was discovered that trans fats may be even more detrimental to your health than saturated fat, the focus has been on getting partially hydrogenated oils out of the diet. But let's not forget about saturated fat, the bulk of which comes from full-fat dairy products, butter, some vegetable oils, and meat, and which is still a health threat because it raises LDL ("bad") cholesterol levels. (Trans fats also raise LDLs and lower HDLs, the "good" cholesterol you want more of.) In fact, the American Heart Association (AHA) just revised its guidelines and dropped the recommended limit on saturated fat in one's diet per day from 10 percent of all fat to 7 percent.

The guidelines we get from health organizations like the AHA are helpful, but don't feel that you have to work the numbers by sitting in your kitchen with a calculator. By switching to nonfat or 1 percent dairy products as you did in Phase Two, you've already removed much of the saturated fat from your diet. Taking out the high-fat protein sources such as certain forms of red meat, pork, and dark-meat poultry (see the chart opposite) are going to whittle it down even further so that your saturated fat intake falls within the AHA guidelines. (The Best Life Meal Plans starting on page 167 are excellent examples of a diet low in both saturated and trans fat.)

There are, of course, also weight-loss and weight-maintenance reasons to remove high-fat meats from your diet: their calorie counts are exponentially higher than those of their lean counterparts. You can reduce the fat on some cuts of meat by cutting off all the visible fat and removing the skin from poultry, but your best strategy is to start with cuts that are naturally lean. Use the chart to help you.

Anything Goes Only High-Fat Meats	Leaner Alternatives
Ground beef	Ground beef, 90% lean or higher; ground turkey—this comes in a variety of fat levels, some of which are ground with the skin on. Look for ground turkey that has no more than 8 g fat and 2.5 g saturated fat per 4 ounces raw turkey.
Rib roasts, porterhouse steaks, brisket, T-bones, and chuck roasts	Flank steak; any cut with the word *loin* in it, such as sirloin or tenderloin (filet mignon is beef tenderloin); and any cut with the word *round* in it (such as top round). Make sure the meat is completely trimmed of fat and that there's little marbling (veins of fat running through the cut).
Veal rib chops, loin chops	Top round, leg cutlet
Pork ribs, ground pork, shoulders, and butts	Cured ham (especially those marked lean or extra lean), pork cutlets, and pork tenderloin
Pork sausage and bacon	Turkey and chicken sausage and turkey bacon
Ground lamb, rack of lamb, loin, and loin chops. (These tend to be lower in fat than beef, but higher than other cuts.)	Leg of lamb and lamb (hind) shank
Sandwich meats like salami, bologna, mortadella, and roast beef	White-meat turkey or chicken
Beef hot dogs	Turkey and vegetarian dogs

WHAT TO EAT INSTEAD: LEANER MEATS, SEAFOOD, EGGS, SOY PRODUCTS

LEAN MEATS: For just about every fatty meat you love, there's a leaner alternative. The chart above provides you with those alternatives and tells you which meats fall into the Anything Goes category.

SEAFOOD: Fish has always been on the top of my list of lean, high-quality protein sources. It's an essentially healthy food that's not only low in calories, but can also be rich in omega-3 fatty acids. But I have to admit that I'm worried about the quality of seafood these days. As pollution has ravaged our waterways, the quality of seafood has gone down; many fish and shellfish now contain polychlorinated biphenyls (PCBs), dioxin, and mercury. Some farmed fish are safer to eat, but it depends on how they are farmed. Farmed fish have been known to accumulate toxins, and some are not farmed in environmentally responsible ways. Also, some types of seafood are overfished, putting the species in danger—another issue you may want to take into account.

While the jury is still out on how harmful the contaminants contained in fish actually are, it's wise to err on the side of caution and limit your intake of seafood, which is why I've also recommended that you take an omega-3 fatty acid supplement. The AHA's recommendation is to eat fish at least twice a week, especially those rich in omega-3s like mackerel, lake trout, sardines, and salmon. I'm more wary. While I still eat fish about once a week, I try to avoid those species that are known to be contaminated or are on the endangered list. For instance, I don't eat canned white (albacore) tuna anymore because most brands of this fish contain mercury (though some groups of researchers believe that the levels are low enough to be harmless and that the benefits of eating tuna outweigh the risks). Instead, if I do eat tuna, I've switched to the "chunk light" kind. I also try to eat wild salmon instead of farmed salmon, though it's a splurge at almost twice the price of the farmed variety. Alaskan salmon, fresh or in the can, is always a safe choice because Alaska has outlawed fish farming, and canned salmon is high in calcium.

The fish story can be very confusing. One type of red snapper may be a good choice while another caught in a different area of the world is overfished, and it's not always possible to know where the fish you're buying is coming from. I think we should all just try to do the best we can, and I'll help you by continuing to update you on seafood issues on my website. You can also get more information from the Monterey Bay Aquarium's Seafood Watch website (mbayaq.org/cr/seafoodwatch.asp) and the Oceans Alive site (www.oceansalive.org/eat.cfm), both of which have comprehensive information about which type of seafood is safe and is gathered in environmentally sensitive ways.

Anything Goes Only

Fish & chips

Fried seafood

Breaded seafood

Fish with butter sauce

EGGS: Eggs are one of the best sources of high-quality protein around. They also contain some important B vitamins as well as the antioxidant selenium. Some egg producers are now also feeding their chickens diets rich in omega-3 fatty acids and vitamin E; eggs from these producers are high in both nutrients.

You may be wondering why I'm recommending eggs, since they are so high in cholesterol. They are, but, for most people, it's largely the saturated fat and not the cholesterol in food that raises blood cholesterol, and eggs have moderate amounts of saturated fat. One egg, for instance, has approximately 1.5 g of saturated fat, about the same as an ounce of 90 percent fat-free beef, and much less than the 6 g of saturated fat in an ounce of cheddar and other full-fat cheeses.

There are some people with high blood cholesterol who are sensitive to cholesterol in foods. If you've been unable to bring down your cholesterol with a diet low in saturated fat and cholesterol, you could be cholesterol sensitive. In that case, consider eating only the whites of eggs (all the dietary cholesterol of eggs is contained in the yolk, as are certain nutrients like vitamin E). Alternatively, just lower the number of yolks that you use. One yolk is about equal in volume to two egg whites, so, for example, if you want to make a three-egg omelet, use one whole egg and four egg whites. While you'll use up your carton faster, eggs are still a relatively inexpensive source of protein, and it's worth the small cost it takes to produce a healthier dish.

For too long, eggs have been considered just a breakfast food, but I think egg dishes like omelets and frittatas are great for lunch and dinner, too. Hard-boiled eggs make a healthy snack and are easy to make. Just boil some up on Sunday and you can have easy-to-grab snacks for the week.

SOY PRODUCTS: The mention of soy once turned some people off, but soy has now so infiltrated the American market that, while I suggest it, many people are already eating it in some capacity. Although it was once only beloved by vegetarians, the more we learn about soy's health benefits—the most prominent one being that it reduces the risk of heart disease—the more it makes sense for nonvegetarians to incorporate this low-calorie protein source into their diet.

If you're among the uninitiated, let me tell you why soy foods are winning over fans. Soybeans, from which tofu and other soy foods are derived, have very little fat and no saturated fat. They contain compounds called isoflavones that may help lower the risk of cancer as well as protect against heart disease. The research on isoflavones shows that getting them naturally through soy foods is healthful, but that too many isoflavones may be too much of a good thing—the estrogen-like properties of isoflavones have some experts worried that too much could promote breast cancer (this is another instance where the jury is still out). For now, avoid soy foods that add extra isoflavones, and don't take isoflavones in supplement form.

Tofu is one of the easiest of soy foods to warm up to. It has virtually no taste, so it will take on the flavor of any herbs, spices, or sauces with which you pair it. It also comes in different textures, from soft and silky to firm and chewy. Many markets now sell seasoned tofu, which is convenient and delicious thrown into salads and stir-fries. Edamame—unprocessed soybeans available in or out of the pod—is another soy food that's easy to love. You can buy edamame frozen in many supermarkets, and they're wonderful as a snack (it takes just five minutes in boiling water to cook them) or tossed into salads and stir-fries.

Soymilk is another good way to get high-quality protein into your diet. You can use it as a substitute for cow's milk; just remember that not all soymilks contain calcium or vitamin D, nutrients which occur naturally in dairy products. Look for soymilks that have been fortified, and always shake the carton well before using the soymilk because the vitamins don't adhere well to the soy and fall to the bottom of the carton. Smoothies are an easy way to incorporate soy into your diet; check the recipe section for some soy smoothies.

SUGAR AND SWEETS

For many people, sweets made with lots of refined white sugar or high-fructose corn syrup are the hardest foods to give up. We are, after all, hard-wired to desire sweet tastes, and if you're used to eating a lot of highly refined sugary foods, there is a good chance that it has even reset your appetite mechanisms, making you crave sweets even more.

The Best Life Diet is not a sugar-free diet; I believe that there's a place for sweets in a healthy diet as long as you consider them a treat, not a dietary staple, and try to make the majority of your sweet choices have some nutritional value. Sugary foods tend to contain few (if any) other nutrients, and let's face it, many sweets are also high in fat—and not the healthful kind. But there is also a whole category of sweet foods that actually do have nutritional value.

If you're devoted to chocolate-chip cookies or like to have a candy bar once in a while, you can use your Anything Goes calories to indulge in them. Otherwise, try to restrict your intake of added sugars to the recommendations on pages 134–136. By added sugars I mean all forms of it (your body treats them all the same way), including refined white sugar, raw sugar, high-fructose corn syrup, corn syrup, fructose, fruit juice sweetener (which is fruit juice boiled down to a thick syrup), honey, maple syrup, molasses, or any other caloric sweeteners added to foods. I'm not referring to naturally occurring sugar in fruit, dried fruit, milk, or plain yogurt (though flavored yogurts have added sugar, too). You'll find sugar not only in obvious places such as pastries and candy, but also in foods you're less likely to think of as sweets, such as some peanut butters and condiments like ketchup and salad dressing.

Similar to what happens with full-fat dairy and salty foods, if you eat fewer sugary foods, you won't desire them so much, and you can actually lose your taste for them over time. That's exactly what you want to happen. The Best Life Diet is a way of eating for a lifetime; the point is not just to resist certain foods for a while, but to change what you crave and what foods give you satisfaction.

Anything Goes Only
Look at the packaging; a sweet food is an Anything Goes treat if a product has:

▶ more than 8 g of sugar (two teaspoons),

▶ a sweetener as one of its first three ingredients, or

- either no sources of naturally occurring sugar (such as the sugar found in fruit or milk) or those sources are way down on the ingredient list.

Anything Goes foods will generally include:

- Maple syrup (all natural *and* maple-flavored)

- Honey

- Jams, jellies, and preserves

- Sweetened beverages like lemonade, energy drinks, and punches

- Sugar in your coffee or tea

- Corn, banana, and carrot breads

- Most commercial muffins

- Candy

- Chocolate

- Cookies

- Cake and other pastries

- Granola bars with more than 12 g sugar

- Non–whole wheat graham crackers

WHAT TO EAT INSTEAD: FRUIT, LOW-SUGAR SWEETS WITH NUTRITIONAL VALUE

Having a piece of fruit is a great way to appease your sweet tooth, especially if the fruit is fresh and in season. But frozen fruit not frozen in syrup can also be very satisfying. I'm surprised at how the array of frozen fruits has grown. It's not just berries anymore; you can also buy frozen mango and even rhubarb. (Cascadian Farm has a great organic selection.) When you don't have fresh fruit on hand, frozen fruit is terrific in smoothies, or stewed and served with a dollop of yogurt on top. Frozen fruit straight from the bag is a cool treat on a hot day. You'll find an array of fruit desserts in

THE SKINNY ON SUGAR SUBSTITUTES

Sugar substitutes do help with weight loss; sugar substitutes don't help with weight loss. Sugar substitutes are harmless; sugar substitutes are unhealthy. The information on sugar substitutes—or as they're often called, zero-calorie artificial sweeteners—like Splenda, aspartame (Equal or NutraSweet), saccharin (Sweet 'N Low), and Acesulfame K is so conflicting that it can make your head spin. What's the truth?

I can only tell you what I know from looking at all of the available evidence. As far as safety goes, there are no long-term human studies on these food additives, so it's difficult to tell whether or not they have any lasting harmful effects. Currently, they are still considered safe by the FDA. Other health watchdog organizations such as the Center for Science in the Public Interest (www.cspinet.org) have given the nod to some of the artificial sweeteners, like Splenda, but not to all of them. I'm going to continue to monitor the science on both sides of the sugar-substitute debate, and you can watch for updates on my website as news comes in.

Whether or not sugar substitutes can help you lose weight is an entirely different question. I think that for some people they can, and many of my clients make the choice to keep them in their diet. I personally don't like the taste of sugar substitutes, so when I want something sweet, I eat something made with fruit or even real sugar. Being very active helps me get away with it. But I realize that if you can't afford the calories and feel that only something sweet will satisfy you, sugar substitutes can help. Most people have grown up with and become accustomed to very sweet foods, which makes it hard to drop them out of their diet overnight. Sugar substitutes can help you bridge the gap while taking out the calories that are preventing you from losing weight.

Foods and beverages that contain sugar substitutes sometimes say so right up front or are called *diet, light* (or *lite*), or *sugar-free.* If you do decide to consume foods or beverages that contain sugar substitutes, be judicious about it. Part of working toward the diet that's going to allow you to keep weight off is changing your taste preferences; having artificially sweetened foods and drinks all day long isn't going to help you lose your taste for sugar. While ultimately the healthiest diet is a diet that's built on all-natural foods free from any type of additives, including sugar substitutes, I know that it's not always easy to eat perfectly and that change doesn't happen overnight. Work toward having the most wholesome diet possible, letting sugar substitutes help you along when necessary, but keeping them to a minimum.

the recipe section of this book. Other great fruit desserts that you can buy or make are all-fruit popsicles, granitas (a frozen dessert made with fruit, a little sugar, and ice), and sorbets.

Although it's taken for granted that desserts are nutritionally empty, that need not be the case. Many sweets can actually help you fulfill your daily recommendations for vitamins, minerals, and fiber. There's a big difference, for instance, between a container of sweetened low-fat fruit yogurt and a dish of frozen yogurt. The former contains much more calcium and has live and active cultures that may keep your digestive tract healthy. Likewise, a dessert such as the Roasted Peaches with Ricotta and Almonds (page 266) or a fruit crisp made with oats (see the Triple-Berry Granola Crisp on page 268) offers you antioxidants, fiber, and healthy fat, while a piece of lemon pound cake or an éclair offers you none of these.

Whenever possible, make the sweets you're going to eat yourself, and when you buy premade ones from the market, check the nutrition facts panel to see how many grams of sugar they contain (see page 125 for your sugar allowance), what the trans fat count is, and if there is anything notably healthy, such as fiber or protein, in the mix. For instance, Slim-Fast Optima Snack Bars satisfy a sweet tooth, but also cover about one-quarter of your daily calcium needs. One note of caution: *low sugar* or *no sugar* doesn't necessarily mean low or no calories, so check the nutrition label to see what you're getting. Also check to see if *sugar-free* means the product contains artificial sweeteners or sugar alcohols, which it often does. (See page 135 for my thoughts on artificial sweeteners.)

Finally, if you know sweets are your weakness, don't keep them on hand. I often hear the excuse "I need to keep cookies in the house for my kids." Do you? Some families go out for an ice cream cone or visit a bakery as a special treat. That approach teaches kids that sweets are not a regular part of everyday dining. Another option is to buy sweets in small, portion-controlled quantities so that if you do want to have them in the house for your family, you can hand your kids something like a prepackaged 100-calorie bag of animal cookies. This will help everyone in your household—including you if you feel the need to indulge—moderate the amount of sweets eaten.

Anything Goes Only

> Fruit desserts
>
> Low-sugar cakes, cookies, and pastries
>
> Canned fruit in syrup
>
> Fruit-only and regular jams and preserves

REFINED GRAINS

In Phase Two, you took white bread out of your diet. Now I'd like you to continue to add whole grains to your diet. Your diet doesn't have to be 100 percent whole grains, but try to make it at least 75 percent. Leave cereals and crackers made from refined grains and white rice behind, and begin working their whole grain counterparts into your day. Buy whole wheat flour, such as Gold Medal Stone Ground Whole Wheat Flour or Arrowhead Mills Whole Wheat Flour. And don't just think *whole wheat*; there is a variety of whole grains out there. While all whole grains share some nutritional attributes like fiber, they each have different healthful properties, so incorporating a variety of different whole grains into your diet will expand the range of nutrients you consume. Look for products already made with a variety of whole grains (things like quinoa pasta or brown rice cakes), or buy them plain and use them as side dishes and in soups and stews. If you live in a place where the selection of whole grains is slim, check the Internet. Bob's Red Mill (no relation!) is a terrific mail-order resource for whole grains and whole grain flours as well as for beans, seeds, and baking mixes (www.bobsredmill.com).

Here are a few different whole grains you may want to try:

Barley: Hulled barley, which is a whole grain, is best, but pearl barley, even though it has the bran removed, is still a good choice because barley's fiber and many of its nutrients are contained in the entire grain. Some canned soups and breads contain whole grain barley, and you can also buy it plain and cook it up as a side dish.

Brown rice: Aside from buying brown rice packaged on its own for cooking as a side dish, you can now find it as the main ingredient in crackers, rice cakes, chips, cereals (hot and cold), pasta, and even rice milk. Try brown basmati and other fragrant varieties of brown rice (Lundberg Family Farms has a number of options). If you don't have the forty-five minutes it takes to cook brown rice, precooked frozen brown rice or brown rice in a shelf-stable pouch is a wonderful (and still nutritious) time-saver.

Buckwheat groats: You can buy this nutty-tasting grain in its whole form or ground as flour. Look for buckwheat pancake mixes and the side dish kasha, which is made from buckwheat groats.

Bulgur: A form of cracked wheat, this is the base for tabbouleh, a Middle Eastern salad often found in the refrigerated section of markets (tabbouleh mixes are available in supermarkets, too). The finely cut type of bulgur is best for tabbouleh, and the coarser cuts make a great stand-in for rice and are cooked basically the same way.

Millet: While just becoming better known here, this grain is a staple in India and other countries. Millet has a mild flavor and is sometimes mixed with other grains or toasted before cooking. Check out the recipe for Curried Chicken, Apple, and Toasted Millet Salad on page 221.

Oats: Oats are rich in soluble fiber, a type of fiber associated with lowering cholesterol. Oats are generally always whole grain, so if you see them on the label (or if you see oat bran), you can feel confident that you're getting the real deal. A great source of oats is, of course, oatmeal, but there are also cold cereals such as Cheerios and Cascadian Farm Organic Purely O's, as well as breads that contain oats.

Quinoa: Pronounced *keen-wah,* this crunchy grain is high in protein and used to make some varieties of pasta and hot and cold cereals. It's also good as a side dish; try it as a change from rice or pasta. See page 260 for Quinoa with Corn, Peppers, and Cilantro.

Whole wheat couscous: Couscous isn't actually a grain; it's a quick-cooking form of pasta made from wheat. While refined forms of couscous have been around for years, whole grain versions are now also hitting the market. It's often served as a side dish and is great with a vegetable stew spooned on top. Fantastic Foods makes a whole wheat couscous, sold nationwide (www.fantasticfoods.com), as does Casbah (www.casbahnaturalfoods.com).

Wild rice: Wild rice isn't particularly high in fiber like other grains, but it's rich in protein, iron, and B vitamins. You can mix it with brown rice to make a nice side dish or grain salad.

There are many ways to work more whole grains into your diet. I personally am a big fan of cereal, and I mix several kinds together so I get a few different kinds of grains (see my cereal mixes in the recipe section on pages 193–194). I am happy to say, though, that cereal and bread, once the only whole grain foods that were easy to find, are now just two of several really terrific whole grain choices on the market. Here are some others to look for. For even more ideas and choices, check my website.

MORE WHOLE GRAIN CHOICES

Whole grain pretzels

Air-popped and low-fat popcorn such as Pop Secret's 94 Percent Fat Free Popcorn (if your popcorn isn't labeled *low-fat,* include it in your Anything Goes calories)

Brown rice sushi

100 percent whole grain bagels and English muffins

Whole wheat tortillas

Whole grain soups (based on barley, wild rice, or whole wheat pasta)

Brown rice chips and cakes

Whole grain crackers

Whole grain waffles

Frozen pizza with whole grain crust

Whole grain cereals

BUYING THE BEST FOOD POSSIBLE

The purpose of the Best Life Diet is to help you lose weight as well as to help you live a healthier life. Part of that includes not only reducing your calorie intake, but also reducing your intake of pesticides and chemical additives. You don't have to have an absolutely pure diet to be healthy; however, it's a good idea to buy organic foods and other foods that have been produced conscientiously whenever you can. Organic foods—the label should read *certified organic*—are those that are produced using standards set forth by the USDA. Those standards stipulate that no pesticides, artificial fertilizers, and, if an animal product, no antibiotics or hormones be used to produce the food. Some foods are labeled *all-natural,* which can indicate that they do not contain chemical additives. But it's a vague term. Look for foods that have a short ingredients list (an indication that the food isn't bolstered with additives) and that do not include artificial flavors or dyes.

Both organic and all-natural foods are becoming more widely available, and that's a good thing. I try to buy as many organic foods as possible and support the efforts of farmers and producers who are committed to cleaning up the environment and producing healthier food. Two of my favorite organic companies whose products carry the Best Life Diet seal of approval are Cascadian Farm and Muir Glen.

The downside is that some organic and natural foods can be more expensive than their less wholesome counterparts, though the prices seem to be coming down as availability is widening. If you're concerned about your budget, consider this: what were you spending before you began this diet? If you were eating out often and buying plenty of convenience foods, with the Best Life Diet you could now be saving some money; why not use some of those savings to buy high-quality organic or natural products? If that's a financial burden, another approach may be to buy only certain organic foods—say, fresh fruits and vegetables but not organic breads or pastas. (If you can't find organic, don't let that stop you from eating lots of fruits and vegetables. The benefits still far outweigh the potential risks. Studies show you can wash off nearly all the pesticide residues by thoroughly washing conventionally grown produce under running water.)

If your problem is that you can't find all-natural and organic foods in your area, consider mail-ordering certain products—grains and beans, in particular, are easy to order via mail. I also recommend visiting a local farmers' market if you have one nearby. Organic and nonsprayed produce (which usually means the farmer doesn't use pesticides but hasn't gone to the trouble and expense of getting certified) tends to be a little cheaper at farmers' markets because it's sold directly to you; there's no middleman driving up the cost. But this is only one of many reasons to patronize farmers' markets. The food at these markets tends to be fresher (sometimes it's picked that very morning), which means it will have more nutrients (some vitamins diminish while produce is shipped and sits on store shelves) and it's going to taste better. Because farmers don't have to worry about how well their fruits are going to fare while transported across the country, they can allow them to ripen on the tree or vine (riper foods are more fragile), which enables them to develop a more complex flavor. The best thing about farmers' markets is that they inspire you to eat more produce. Just taking a spin around the market and seeing all those gorgeous rows of fresh vegetables, fruits, and herbs are enough to make you want to rush right home and toss them all into a salad!

Add More Wholesome Foods to Your Diet

I could have called this section "Add More Healthful Foods to Your Diet," because that is what you're going to do. But for many people "healthful foods" sounds punishing, as if having to eating them is like being put in dietary jail. That's not a fitting description for the foods that I want you to add to your diet; these foods are flavorful and satisfying.

Of course, most healthful foods are not infused with the intense (and often artificial) flavors that most unhealthy foods are, but there are so many companies now making wonderful-tasting, nutritious foods as well as cooks who are coming up with terrific (and easy) ways to turn healthful ingredients into fantastic meals. That's what the recipes and product recommendations in this book are for, and I hope that you'll use them to help you transition into thoroughly healthy eating. And there's more where those recipes and recommendations came from. I created my website with the intention that it would be an ongoing resource for finding and making great food. The Best Life Team will be testing, tasting, and shopping the grocery store aisles to keep you informed of what's new and worth trying.

In the following sections, I'm going to talk about *all* the wholesome foods you should be adding to your diet. Sure, you know that you should be eating more fruits and vegetables, whole grains, beans, and other nutritious foods, but I want to give you more specifics and tell you about some of the best ways to eat them from a weight-control, good-health, *and* flavor-conscious standpoint. If healthy eating is an acquired taste, you're going to develop a taste for it relatively quickly by following these guidelines.

VEGETABLES

With all of the talk about high-protein diets in recent years, the importance of vegetables has been shoved to the side. That's really a shame, because vegetables are the best foods you can eat for weight loss and good health. They're one of the best sources of disease-fighting phytonutrients; are water- and fiber-packed, which makes them extremely filling; and, when prepared properly, can't be beat for their terrific, fresh flavor. Hundreds of studies of populations all over the world show that people who eat the most vegetables (and fruits) have the lowest risk of cancer.

One of the goals of the Best Life Diet is to get you to eat more vegetables. In fact, your goal should be to make vegetables the food you eat the most. Depending on your activity level, you should eat at least four servings of vegetables a day (see page 126 for serving sizes); but if you eat them without added fat, you can (and should) eat lots more. You'll see that it's not that hard: try a large salad filled with several different kinds of vegetables. The only vegetables you may want to go easy on are potatoes, corn, and peas. Because they're as starchy (and about as caloric) as grains, you should count them as grain servings.

Some vegetables have more to offer than others. Generally, the deeper the color of the vegetable, the more nutrients it will have. The vibrant colors of sweet potatoes, carrots, spinach, chard, tomatoes, and red peppers are indicators of large amounts of vitamins and phytonutrients. But each color is also associated with a string of different nutrients, so your best strategy is to include vegetables (and fruit, for that matter) of varying colors in your diet to help you cover all your nutrient bases. (See the color-guide chart on page 147 for more information.)

Another category of vegetables you should be including in your diet is the cruciferous family: broccoli, cauliflower, Brussels sprouts, kale, collards, mustard greens, rutabagas, and turnips. These vegetables have been linked to cancer prevention, and some of them, mostly kale, collards, and mustard greens, are also good sources of calcium.

I also recommend bolstering your diet with mushrooms, a good source

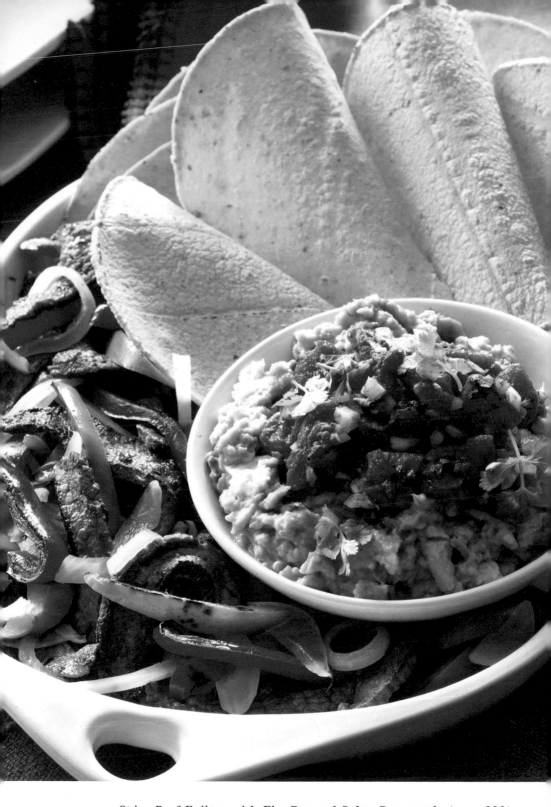

Spicy Beef Fajitas with Fire-Roasted Salsa Guacamole (page 232)

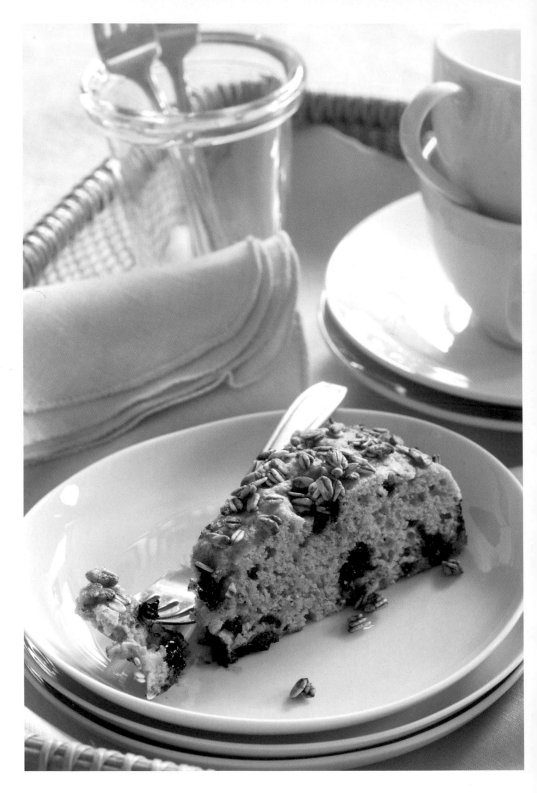

Blueberry Yogurt Coffee Cake (page 265)

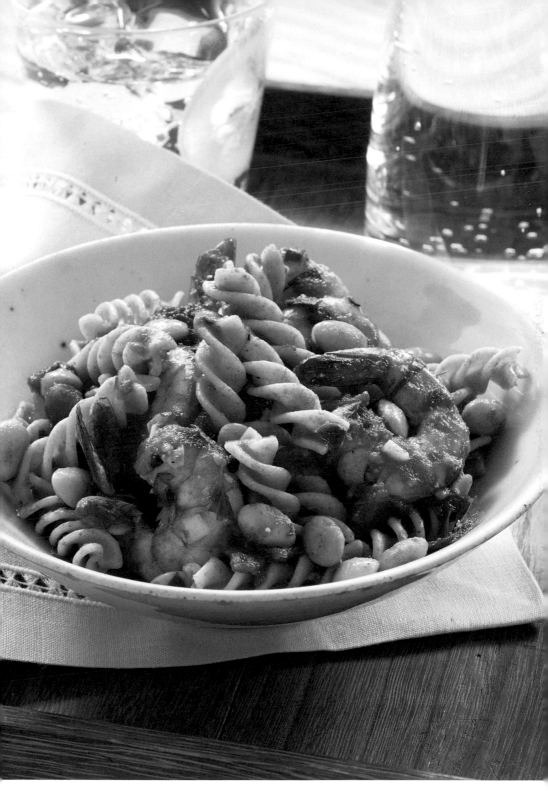

Shrimp and Edamame Rotini (page 250)

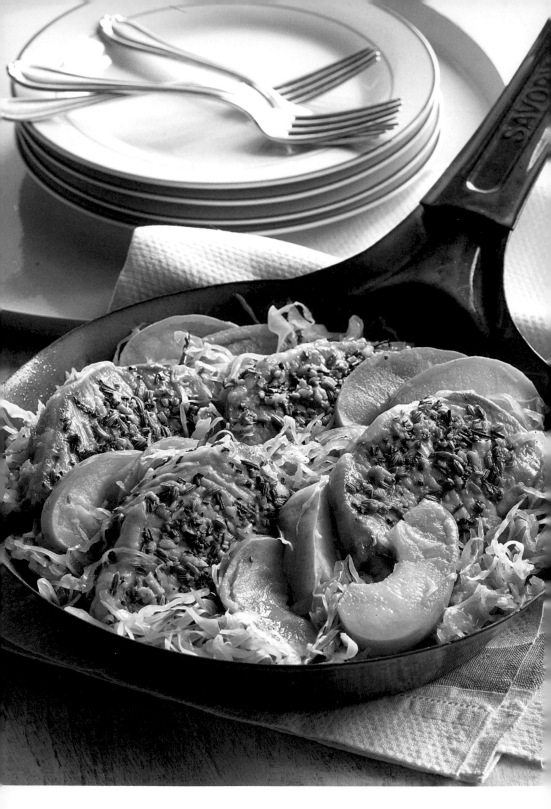

Pork Chop and Cabbage Bake (page 239)

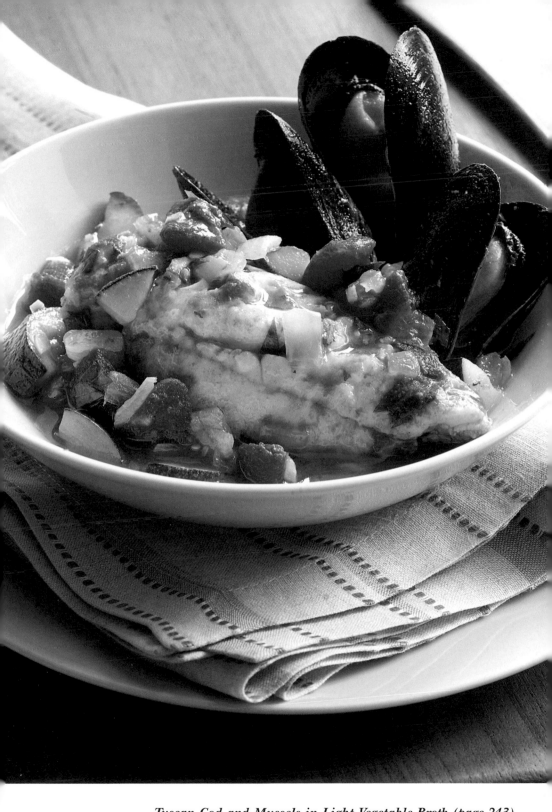

Tuscan Cod and Mussels in Light Vegetable Broth (page 243)

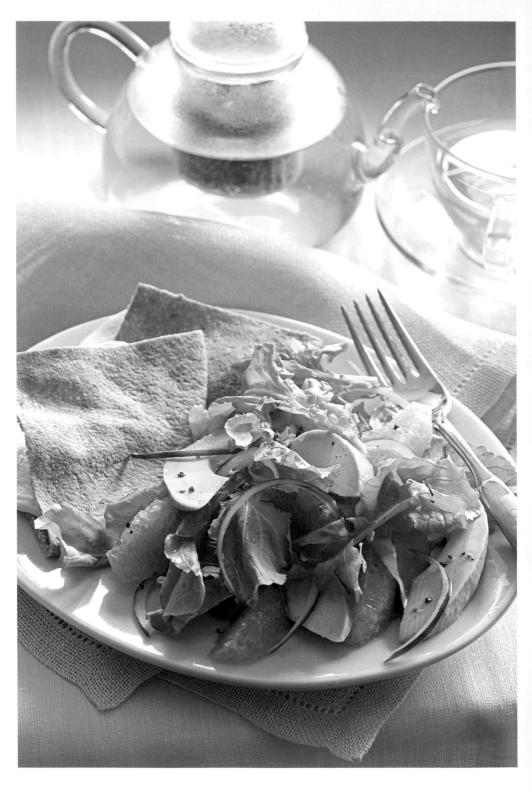

Arugula, Grapefruit, and Avocado Salad (page 211)
with whole wheat pita and fresh mozzarella (Meal Plans, page 166)

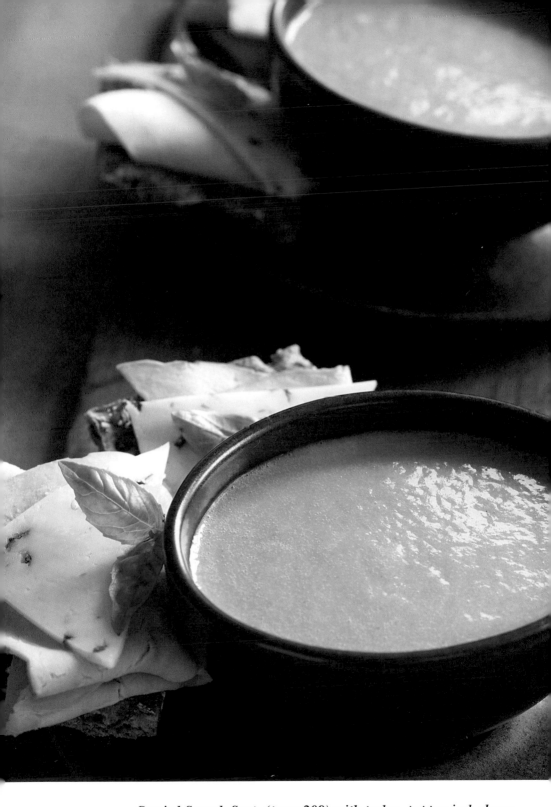

*Curried Squash Soup (page 209) with turkey, pepper jack cheese,
and fresh basil leaves on Wasa crispbread (Meal Plans, page 163)*

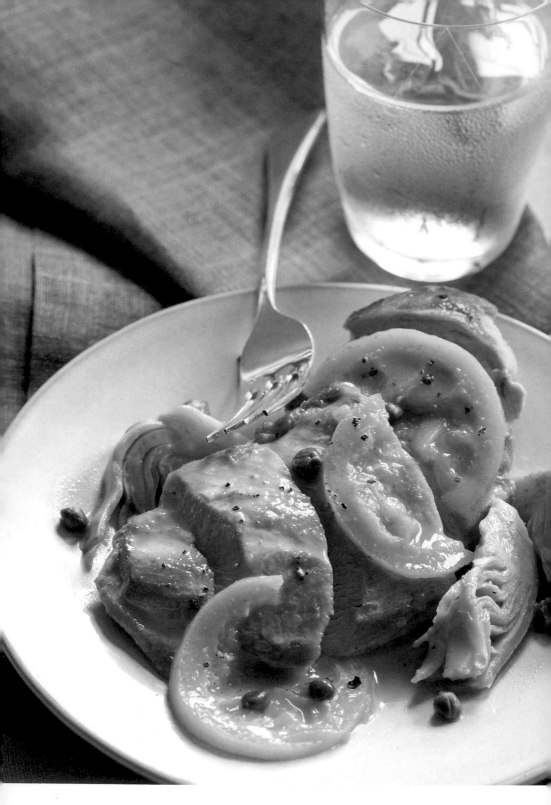

Chicken with Artichokes and Melted Lemons (page 234)

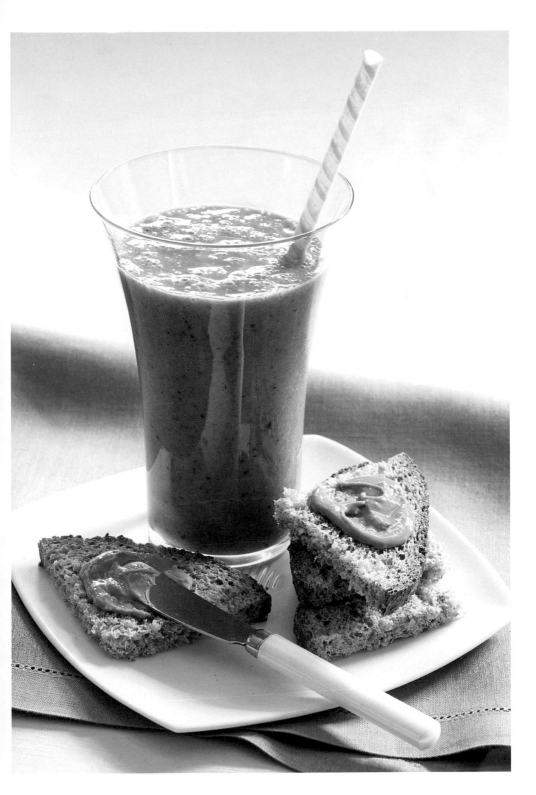

Strawberry-Orange Smoothie (page 199) with peanut butter on
Ezekiel 4:9 Organic Sprouted Whole Grain Bread (Meal Plans, page 166)

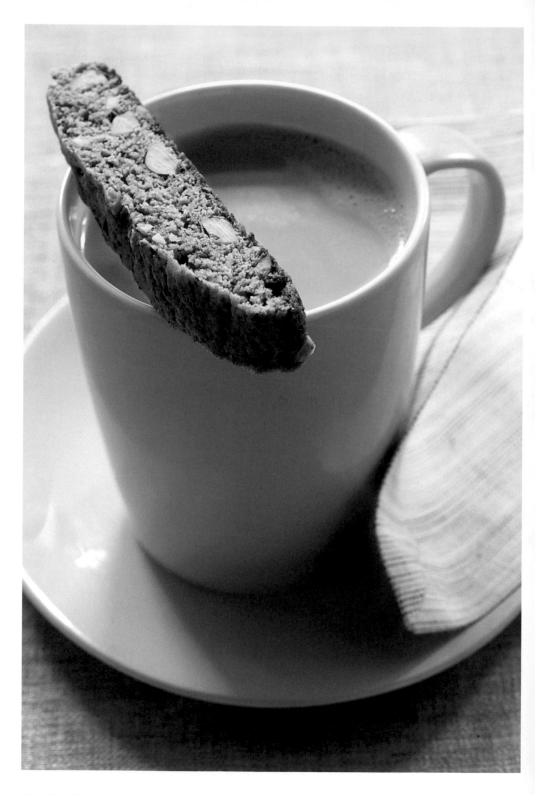

Vanilla Caramel Truffle Latte (page 271)
with Hazelnut Biscotti (page 269)

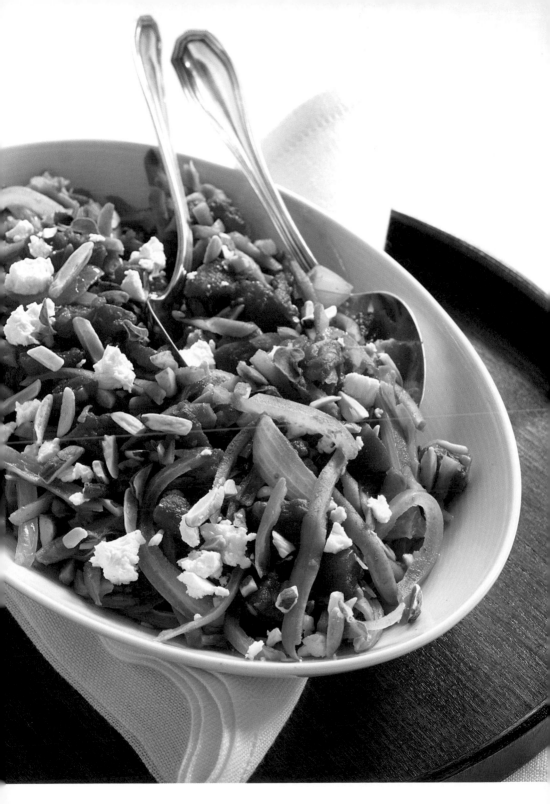

Green Beans with Tomatoes and Feta (page 255)

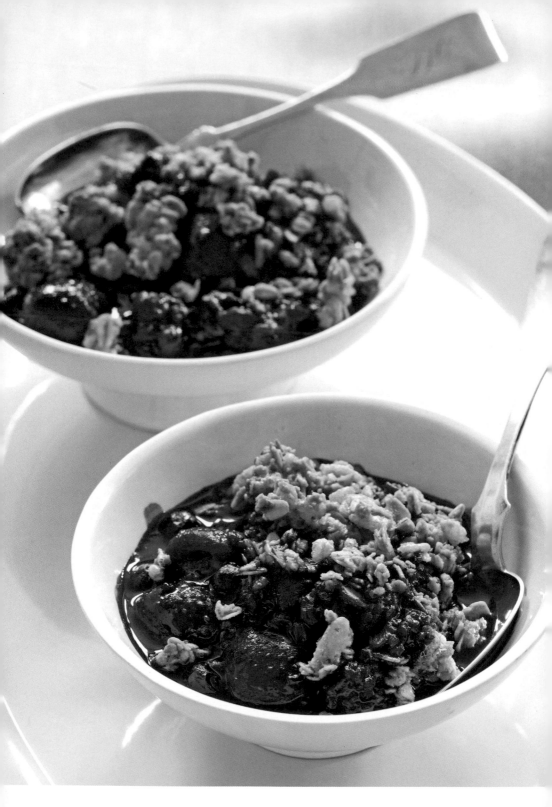

Triple-Berry Granola Crisp (page 268)

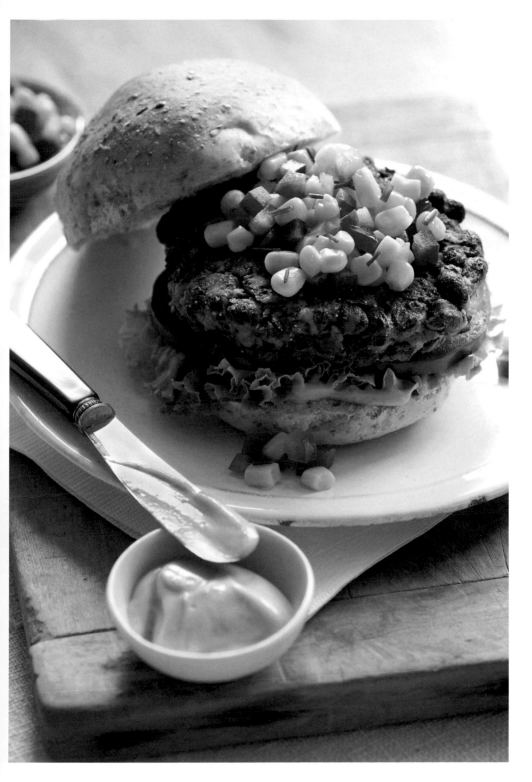

Black Bean Chipotle Burger with Corn Salsa (page 224)

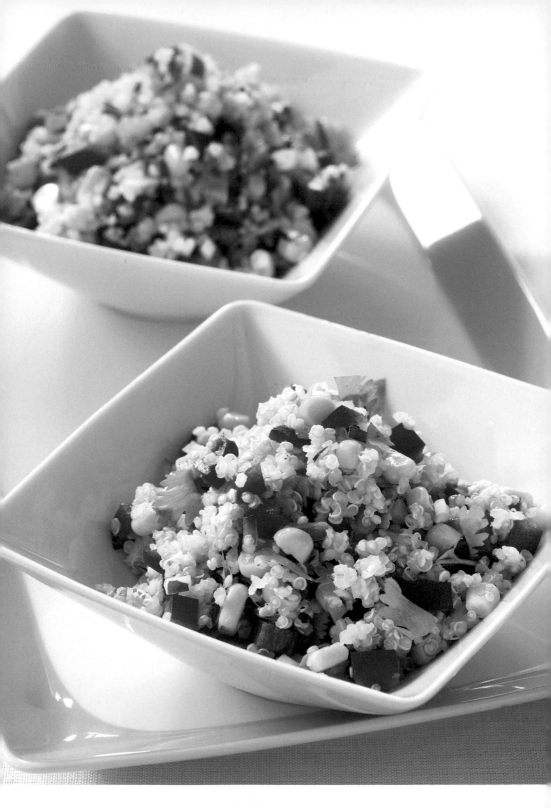

Quinoa with Corn, Peppers, and Cilantro (page 260)

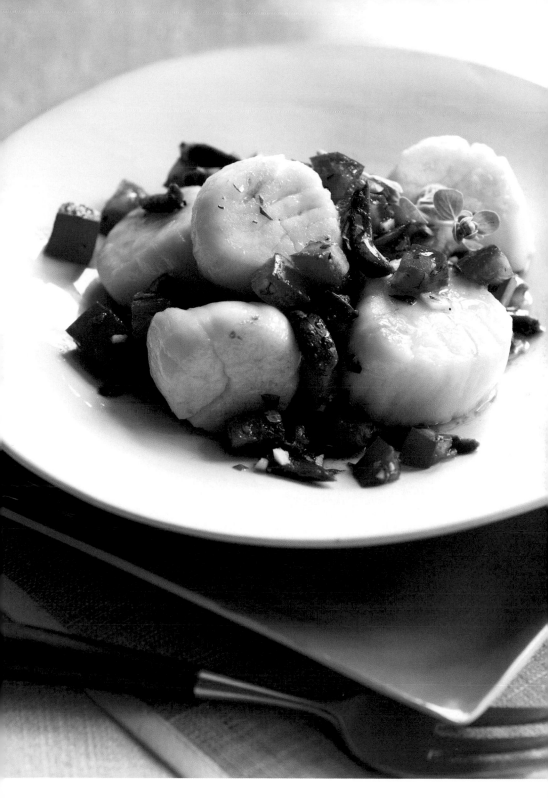

Roasted Scallops with Tomato Salsa (page 245)

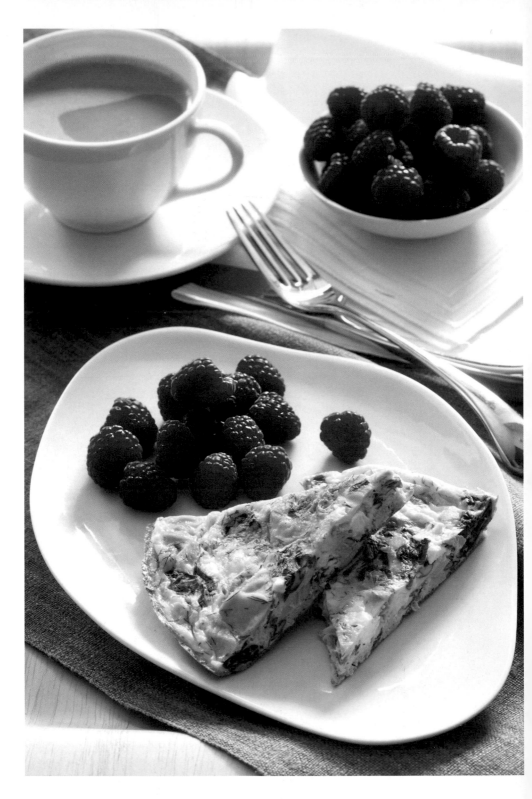

*Salmon and Spinach Frittata (page 200) with berries
and café au lait (Meal Plans, page 189)*

of antioxidants. A study at Penn State University found that mushrooms are a particularly good source of antioxidants called polyphenols.

While vegetables are the natural go-to foods for anyone trying to lose or maintain weight, there's little point in piling your plate high with them if you're going to drown them in fat. Serving vegetables without fat can be a sticking point for some people, especially if you've grown up eating them smothered in cheese or swimming in butter, but there are several good ways to approach that problem. First, while I don't recommend you cook a pot of broccoli coated in cheddar, you don't have to forgo fat totally when you're cooking vegetables. For a long time, steamed (or blanched) vegetables were the only kind anyone trying to lose weight could eat, but I think they actually turned people off to nutritious eating. There's no reason you have to settle for bland veggies: you can put herbs and garlic in the steaming water to give them a bit more flavor. You can also drizzle your portion with a tiny bit of olive oil and add a spritz of fresh lemon juice or sprinkle on a little Parmesan cheese or grated low-fat cheddar after cooking.

You can sauté vegetables as long as you're using just a small amount of fat; a good rule of thumb is to use no more than 1½ teaspoons of olive oil per person. Fat actually helps the body absorb carotenes and other phytonutrients in the vegetables.

Here are some other ways to add variety and flavor and work more vegetables into your diet.

▶ *Roast vegetables:* Roasting gives vegetables a wonderful sweetness and allows you to prepare them with a minimum amount of fat. Toss the vegetables with a touch of olive oil if you like, or use a little balsamic vinegar to add oomph.

▶ *Use broth for extra flavor:* Heat a little olive or other healthy oil in a pan over medium heat. When the oil is hot, toss in chopped vegetables of your choice and let them cook for two to three minutes. Then pour in a cup or so (it doesn't matter how much, because you'll cook it down) of reduced-sodium chicken or vegetable broth. Cover the pan for one to two minutes so the vegetables steam, then remove the lid and continue cooking until the vegetables are completely wilted or tender-crisp.

▶ *Keep frozen vegetables on hand:* Frozen produce can sometimes be even more nutritious than fresh because it's flash frozen right after it's been picked, before its nutrients have a chance to degrade. Fresh produce, on the other hand, can spend days being transported and sitting on supermarket shelves before it arrives at your table. By that time, many nutrients, and in particular carotenes and vitamin C, which are destroyed by light, are lost. Look for frozen vegetables that have 0 or close to 0 mg sodium, and if you choose frozen vegetables with a sauce, check to make sure that it has no more than 350 mg of sodium per serving and no trans fats. Two varieties I like to keep on hand are Green Giant spinach and Cascadian Farm winter squash— it's so easy to just throw them into pasta or soup, and they up the nutritional value of each dish considerably.

▶ *Use healthy dips:* Dip your carrot, celery, and red pepper sticks into low-fat or nonfat ranch dressing.

▶ *Buy preshredded cabbage or coleslaw mix:* Make coleslaw with a light vinaigrette rather than a mayonnaise dressing.

▶ *Try a new vegetable each week:* Some vegetables that often get ignored but are worth sampling include jicama (terrific sprinkled with lime juice and chili powder; adds crunch to salads), hearts of palm (comes in cans and is great sliced into salads), beets (look for them in various colors and try roasting them), Swiss chard (use as you would spinach—look for different color chards, which are beautiful served together), celery root (good cooked and pureed or raw in salads), and radishes (they add some crunch to salads as well as cancer-fighting compounds).

Anything Goes Only

Vegetables in butter, cream, or cheese sauce that have *more* than 3 g fat and 1.5 g saturated fat per serving

Coleslaw or salads in creamy dressing

Baked potatoes with sour cream

French fries

Fried vegetables

VEGETABLE HUNGER STOPPERS: SOUPS AND SALADS

Soups and salads deserve their own special category, because they're great aids for keeping the calories you consume to a minimum. Let's start with soup. Research at Purdue University has shown that people eat fewer calories throughout the day when they have soup for one of their meals. Additionally, the research of Barbara Rolls, PhD, a satiety researcher at Penn State, has shown that having a broth-based soup before a meal can reduce how much you eat at that meal by as much as 100 calories. I think that makes plenty of sense, because hot soup is such a great comfort food in the winter and cold soup is so refreshing in the summer. And both types seem to stick to your ribs, even though it takes very little fat (and therefore not a lot of calories) to make a hearty soup. (I'm excluding cream soups from this discussion because they're usually so high in two things you *don't* want in your diet: saturated fat and cholesterol. When there are so many great noncream soups, you should be able to do without them, but if you feel you must have them, use your Anything Goes calories.)

I also love soups because they make it easy to get in a lot of vegetables (think how many veggies get tossed into your average minestrone) and one pot goes a long way. If you cook up a big batch of soup on Sunday, you'll have plenty of meals for the coming week (even if you set aside some for the freezer), and that is a good way to help ensure that you don't stray from your diet. It's when you come home from a long day and making something healthy to eat seems like a huge effort that you will be vulnerable to dialing up for pizza delivery. When you've got something satisfying like soup in the fridge or freezer, you're going to have a much more healthful and calorie-conscious fallback.

So I encourage you to eat soup regularly either as a starter to a meal or as the meal itself. I'm impressed with how many great soups in cans (and cartons) are now on the market—one of my favorite is Progresso's lentil soup, which is convenient and has a homemade taste. When you're shopping for canned soup, watch out for those that are high in sodium. Canned soups tend to be higher in sodium than most foods, so if you have high blood pressure, you may want to avoid them. If a soup has more than 600 mg of sodium per cup, have no more than just one cup.

I'm almost a little reluctant to bring up salads, because nothing makes you think of the pain of dieting faster than a salad. It used to be that whenever you'd go out to eat and someone ordered a salad, it was a clear sign that that person was trying to lose weight. But it turned out that many of the salads people were eating were even more fattening than the steak and potatoes they were avoiding! The typical chef's salad loaded with meat and cheese has been clocked in at 930 calories and 71 g of fat. A restaurant chicken Caesar salad can have as much as 660 calories and 46 g of fat.

Naturally, I don't recommend that you eat these types of salads. But salads that have lots of leafy greens and vegetables; are dressed moderately; aren't loaded with cheese, meat, croutons, nuts, tuna and chicken salads made with mayonnaise, and other high-fat extras can be a healthful addition to your diet. And like soups, they can help you add a large variety of vegetables to your diet. Rolls's work has also shown that people who started their meal with a salad ate fewer calories overall during the meal, just as when they started with soup.

The healthiest salads start with a good base. Choose darker greens like romaine, arugula, watercress, spinach, and mesclun mix, which have more vitamins and minerals than lighter-colored greens like iceberg lettuce. Then add an array of other vegetables—peppers, tomatoes, radishes, cucumbers, snow peas, artichoke hearts, sprouts, mushrooms, beets, jicama, water chestnuts . . . the sky really is the limit, and the more varied your choices, the more interesting your salad will taste. You don't have to leave out all of the extras completely, but limit them. If you're adding in grated cheddar cheese, avocado, or nuts, include only one tablespoon (two for a meal-size salad) of the item and use a low-fat dressing.

If you're making your own dressing at home, use a flavorful vinegar such as an aged balsamic, sherry, or rice vinegar, which will allow you to reduce the oil in the recipe. Olive oil—especially extra-virgin olive oil—is a natural base for salad dressings, but if you don't like the strong taste, go with a light-tasting olive oil or use canola oil. (Bertolli even has an extralight olive oil.) If you prefer creamy dressings, try substituting non- or lowfat yogurt in recipes that call for mayonnaise. In restaurants, always order dressings on the side, and instead of dumping the whole cup onto your

A Guide to Color-Coded Eating

A fruit's or vegetable's color is a good indicator of the different vitamins, minerals, and phytonutrients it contains. Put a rainbow on your plate, and you're going to cover a lot of your nutrient bases. Here's a color-by-color breakdown.

Fruit/Vegetable Color or Type	Such as . . .	What They Bring to the Table
Green	Asparagus, beet greens, broccoli, Brussels sprouts, collard greens, dandelion greens, green beans, honeydew melon, kale, kiwi, mustard greens, okra, parsley, peas, peppers, spinach, Swiss chard, romaine lettuce, and zucchini.	Lutein and zeaxanthin, powerful antioxidants (especially lutein) linked to reducing risk of two eye diseases: cataracts and macular degeneration, the leading cause of blindness. Many are also good sources of beta-carotene.
White/Green	Artichokes, asparagus, celery, chives, endive, garlic, green pears, mushrooms, onions, and scallions.	Onions, potatoes, and garlic especially are rich in allyl sulfides, which help prevent stomach and colon cancer and may lower cholesterol. Onions are also a good source of quercitin, protecting against cancer and possibly heart disease. The rest contain flavonoids, a large class of phytonutrients linked to preventing heart disease.
Cruciferous (a family of mostly green-white vegetables)	Arugula, bok choy, broccoflower (a broccoli-and-cauliflower hybrid), broccoli, Brussels sprouts, cabbage (all types), cauliflower, collard greens, kale, mustard greens, rutabaga, Swiss chard, turnips, turnip greens, and watercress.	Cancer-fighting compounds called indoles and isothiocyanates.
Yellow/Orange	Apricots, carrots, sweet potatoes, pumpkin, butternut squash, cantaloupe, mangoes, citrus fruit, and peaches.	Bioflavonoids, which may help protect against cancer and heart disease, and vitamin C. Citrus peel contains limonene, which also helps fight cancer. Some have beta- and alpha-carotene, antioxidants that are linked to reducing the risk of cancer and heart disease.
Red	Pink grapefruit, red tomatoes, salsa, tomato-based juices, tomato-based pasta sauce, tomato soup, and watermelon.	Vitamin C and lycopene, a powerful antioxidant linked to protection from cancer and heart disease, give these foods their red color.
Purple/Blue/ Deep Red	Red beets, cherries, cranberries, eggplants, grape juice, plums, prunes, raisins, red apples, red beans, red cabbage, red or purple grapes, red onions, red pears, red wines, and strawberries.	Anthocyanins, a potent group of antioxidants that helps prevent blood clots and may improve brain function.

salad at once, dip the tines of your fork lightly into the dressing, then take a bite. By the salad's end, you'll have used less dressing. At home, use the same technique, or "spray" your salad with dressing; Wish-Bone Salad Spritzers only dispense about 1 calorie per spray.

The following are some other healthy extras that make salads delicious without adding too many calories:

► Fiber-rich legumes like garbanzo beans, kidney beans, or black beans

► Lean meats like turkey, turkey bacon, chicken, baked tofu (available preseasoned at natural food markets and supermarkets), hard-boiled egg whites, tuna, shrimp, or crabmeat

► Chunks or slices of fresh fruits like apples, pears, mandarin oranges, grapefruit, apricots, blueberries, strawberries, mangoes, or pineapples

► Dried fruit like figs, apricots, raisins, cherries, or cranberries (keep it to two tablespoons, since the calories in dried fruit can add up)

Anything Goes Only

Cream soups

Creamy salad dressings (unless they're low-fat)

Caesar salads (unless they're low-fat)

Chef salads

FRUIT

Some people, worried about the amount of sugar in their diets, stop eating fruit. Other people, those who belong to the if-a-little-is-good-a-lot-must-be-better school of thought, eat fruit to their heart's content. Neither one of these tactics is a good idea; finding the middle ground is. You should eat at least two servings of fruit a day, maybe more if you're very active (see the Best Life Diet Guidelines on pages 124–126).

You should also try to vary the fruits you eat just as you vary the vegetables you consume. Grapefruit, for instance, have different nutritional attributes than peaches, which have different attributes than apples, and so on. You'll also get the most health benefits from fruit if you largely stick to eating whole fruit rather than drinking juice. Juice, especially fresh squeezed, does generally contain a good dose of vitamins and phytonutrients; however, it doesn't contain as much fiber as whole fruit (although pulp-filled juices do have some fiber).

Juice contains a lot of sugar, and for that reason, it's a good idea to drink juice in moderation. If you're a real juice lover like me, consider smoothies. Since smoothies (at least the healthiest ones) are made with fruit, not just juice, they can have more fiber and less sugar ounce per ounce. Your best bet, though, is to make smoothies yourself so you know exactly what's in them. (Try out the smoothie recipes on pages 198–199 and 272.) Some restaurants and food outlets add sherbet and frozen yogurt, and not necessarily the low-fat kind, to their smoothies, which drive up the calorie count.

I also suggest you go easy on dried fruit. While it's a great snack, it doesn't have the water content of fresh fruit, and that can make it less filling. And it's so easy to keep putting your hand back in the bag of dried fruit, so ultimately you eat upward of, say, six whole apricots. If you were eating fresh ones, chances are you'd eat a lot fewer. Many varieties of dried fruit also contain sulfites, a preservative. Be wary, too, of fruit rolls. Those that are made solely from fruit and fruit juice are fine, but some have both added sugar and other additives.

When I was a kid, I was always disappointed when we had fruit for dessert. It didn't seem like a real treat. But now that I know there are so many different kinds of fruit and different ways to serve them, I'm happy to see fruit on the table after dinner, especially when it's a type of fruit that's in season. Here are some ways to get more fruit into your diet.

▶ Tropical fruits are so sweet and luscious that they launch fruit flavor into a whole other realm. Try pineapple, mangoes, papayas, passion fruit, kiwi, and guavas (guavas must be very ripe if you want to eat them raw), and if you can't find them fresh, look for frozen chunks, which are great in smoothies. Tropical fruits can be a little more expensive than apples and oranges, but they'll take less of a toll on your wallet, not to mention your body, than a box of cookies.

▸ You'll enjoy fruit so much more if you eat it seasonally. Peaches in winter, usually flown in from faraway places, tend to be hard and flavorless. Plus, if your fruit bowl changes with the seasons, you're less likely to get bored. Go for strawberries in spring; stone fruit, such as peaches, plums, nectarines, and apricots, in summer; apples and pears in the fall; and grapefruit and tangerines in the winter.

▸ One of the great things about our expanding food markets is that we're now seeing a lot of varieties within the families of very familiar fruits. (This is especially true if you shop at farmers' markets.) So if you're used to eating Granny Smith and Red Delicious apples, give Pink Ladies and Fujis a try. Swap Bartlett pears for Bosc and casaba melon for cantaloupe. If you usually buy navel oranges, try Satsuma mandarins, tangelos, blood oranges, and pink grapefruits. Pink and red grapefruit are such a great source of the cancer fighter lycopene—plus a University of Florida College of Medicine study found that adding grapefruit to the diet reduced levels of LDL "bad" cholesterol by 11 percent in sixteen weeks. Studies have also shown that grapefruit lowers triglycerides and may lower the risk of lung cancer. I eat grapefruit just like oranges, peeled and in sections. The more adventurous you are, the more treasures you'll find.

▸ Serve fruit in different ways. Poached pears, baked apples, and fruit salads are a few ways to enjoy fruits instead of straight from the crisper. Puree melons into cold soups and turn peaches and berries into compotes.

Anything Goes Only

Fruit sorbets, ices, and granitas

Fruit crumbles, crisps, buckles, and betties

Fruit leathers with sugar (look for the ones made without sugar, which can be part of your regular diet)

Fruit tarts

Fruit with honey or other sweet sauces

BEANS

I put beans into the super-food category. When I was growing up, my family would have baked beans once in a while, and I'd seen navy bean soup on menus (though I never ate it). And that was basically all I knew about beans. I'm so glad that times have changed, because I've come to enjoy so many different types of beans, from black and pinto to cannellini, fava, and anasazi. Beans are a great lean source of protein and have the added attraction of providing a big hit of fiber, too. I recommend working them into your diet at least a couple times a week, whether in a bean-based soup or chili, rolled up in a wrap or a burrito, combined with pasta or other grains, or just by themselves, eaten the Italian way, with a drizzle of olive oil, a sprinkling of herbs (try fresh chopped rosemary), and a little salt and pepper. Also check out the bean recipes in this book, such as Kale and White Bean Soup (page 204), Whole Wheat Burritos with Black Beans, Brown Rice, Greens, and Corn Salsa (page 228), and Vegetarian Chili (page 251).

It's really not difficult to make beans at home. You simply need to soak the dried beans overnight (or follow the quick-soak directions on the package label), throw them in a pot with water to cover, bring them to a boil, and let them simmer until tender. Toss in a chopped onion and a few mashed cloves of garlic to give them more flavor. The one problem you can run up against with homemade beans is that old beans are very tough and take a long time to cook. Unfortunately, there's no way to tell how old the beans that you're buying are. Try to purchase beans from places that have a good turnover (if there's dust on the package, it's not a good sign), and if you ever see dried beans at a farmer's market, snap them up. They're usually very fresh and cook in no time.

Canned beans are also a great alternative. In fact, I think they're one of the best-tasting canned foods there are. Just make sure to rinse the beans with water before using them to get rid of some of the sodium. You may also look for the no-salt-added and lower-sodium (140 mg or less per half cup) canned beans, a staple of health-food stores that are now showing up in mainstream markets, too.

Healthy Fats

NUTS AND SEEDS

Eating nuts and seeds is another way to get protein into your diet and, perhaps even more important, is a good source of heart-healthy fats. Walnuts, almonds, cashews, peanuts, pecans, pumpkin seeds, sunflower seeds, and flaxseeds are the most nutritious. They are a great addition to your diet, but you really have to be cautious: you can rack up quite a few calories eating nuts and seeds, particularly the ones that have been roasted in oil. The sensory quality of nuts and seeds is such that, once you put your hand into the peanut bowl, it can be hard to stop even if your stomach is telling you it's had enough; about two to four tablespoons of nuts or seeds should be your limit.

There are several ways that you can work nuts and seeds into your diet without overdoing it. One is to use just a sprinkling of them in vegetable salads (sunflower seeds, walnuts, and pecans are particularly good in savory dishes like salads) and fruit salads (try hazelnuts and almonds). Nuts are also good scattered over fruit desserts. Another way to use nuts and seeds is to mix a small amount into your cereal in the morning or to throw some into a stir-fry (peanuts and cashews are great in Asian dishes). Grind up flaxseeds and add them to baked goods or stir them into cereal. If you prefer to eat nuts and seeds as a snack, divide big jars into small snack-size bags (put in one-fourth of a cup of nuts in each) so it's easier to limit your intake. Store nuts and seeds in the freezer, because they don't have a particularly long shelf life and can go rancid.

Using nut and seed butters is a great alternative, and there are many options beyond peanut butter (though peanut butter is a good choice, too). Almond, pistachio, cashew, pumpkin seed, hazelnut, sunflower seed, and soy butters have their own unique flavors. (Brazil nut, cashew nut, and macadamia nut butters are also available, but contain a fair amount of saturated fat.) You can use nut and seed butters on sandwiches, on toast for breakfast, or on whole grain crackers as a snack.

Anything Goes Only

Trail Mix that includes chocolate or carob chips

Sesame candy bars

Fruit and nut bars

Peanut brittle

Candied pecans or other candied nuts

Roasted and salted nuts

Judging Your Success

At this point, you have all the elements of a healthful diet spelled out for you. You can now set your parameters as well as decide the pace at which you want to adopt the changes you choose to make. You can tighten up—or loosen up—the limitations you put on your diet, including your Anything Goes calories. Step back and look at how things are going. If you feel you need to lose more weight, you may want to give yourself fewer Anything Goes calories and/or increase your activity. Readjust those calories and all your dietary choices in order to meet your goals.

Weight loss will be one measure of your success on this program, but the true measure will be whether you've achieved *your* best life. Keep going, savoring and celebrating each small step that you make toward attaining the life you want.

PATIENCE,
PERSEVERANCE,
AND A
POSITIVE ATTITUDE

If you think you can or you think you can't, you're right.
— HENRY FORD

▶ I've been helping people make lifestyle changes for over twenty-five years, and one thing is very clear: changing our behavior is one of the toughest things we can do. Changing how we eat is particularly tough due to our primitive hardwiring. We're born with mechanisms that make us want to eat high-calorie foods—and lots of them!

With the right approach, we can overcome those instincts. The tougher challenge, for some people, is another kind of hardwiring: negative, firmly ingrained attitudes about the world and themselves that were formed when they were very young. So much of our behavior is dictated by how we think, and how we think tends to stay static—unless we consciously try to change it. And that's key: if you're hampered by a negative attitude, you're going to need to think differently. Change your attitude and you can change your life, too.

This program sets out quite a few challenges for you. It asks you to change how active you are, when you eat, what you eat, and what you drink. It also asks you to set about changing the areas of your life that are troubled or in which you are unfulfilled so you will stop turning to food for comfort. You are capable of all of these things, but only if you believe you are. If there's one thing that people who make major—and permanent—changes in their lives have in common, it's a positive outlook. I can't stress how important this is. But you don't have to be born with a glass-is-half-full attitude; you can develop one. It's a thrilling process; the process of positive change can be one of the best experiences of your life if you let it.

Here's what it takes to be the optimistic and confident person you need to be to succeed: Focus on the good things that happen in your life each day rather than the bad. What went right today? What things did you do to benefit yourself? This doesn't mean that you need to avoid thinking about what went wrong; going over what you would have done differently is the best way to learn. But look at those things as something you can work to change, and vow to do better tomorrow.

This is where having a journal can be enormously helpful. Sit down in solitude, in a quiet room, maybe with some soothing music playing and a cup of tea on the table; then write about where in your life you need to make improvements. The perfect time to do this is when you're tempted to eat, because the process can not only distract you from eating, but it can also help you be proactive and positive about the changes you're making. Writing demands that you focus, and that will help you face challenges head-on instead of letting vague thoughts of change hover in the back of your mind. Even if you just have moments of feeling hopeful, capturing them on paper can generate more of these moments. Positive thinking is like a ball rolling downhill: it may start out slowly, but it will gather momentum, inspiring and motivating you to create a better life for yourself.

Having a positive attitude prepares you to take the next steps toward change. Those steps are:

► Make an honest assessment of yourself and what you're willing to change about yourself and your behavior.

► Determine what you need to do to accomplish those changes.

► Muster up the discipline needed to make it all happen.

► Avoid getting discouraged along the way.

Getting discouraged can be hard to avoid. But not if you look at obstacles as opportunities and at challenges as a chance to show your mettle. In other words, take pleasure in persevering; that's what separates those people who keep pushing forward from those who throw in the towel. From what I've observed, people who persevere delight in each small victory. To them, having the inner strength to turn down a piece of cake at a party is cause for celebration. They feel good about themselves for their self-discipline, and their self-esteem, along with their motivation, grows. Perseverance is born out of affirming each small accomplishment along the way to a larger goal. That's what is going to help you develop the optimism you need to succeed.

Not allowing yourself to be discouraged and acknowledging your small victories is also what's going to help you have the patience to see this program through. Dramatic change doesn't happen in one day or even one month, and that can be discouraging if you're used to (and long for) immediate gratification. It's easier, though, to be patient when you feel as though you're reaping some kind of reward for your efforts; that's why it's so important to enjoy the process of positive change rather than focusing on the end result. Find joy in each triumph, big or small. Don't take for granted turning down a piece of cake, eating a healthful breakfast, or going for a walk at lunch—or any of the small but significant efforts you make as part of your commitment to this program. All of them count, and with continued patience, perseverance, and a positive attitude, they're all going to add up to a big payoff.

If there is any secret to success, it's this: Be honest with yourself and those around you. Take responsibility for your actions and your life. Think of the commitments you make to yourself as sacred, and honor them in the way that you honor your commitments to other people. Identify what it is you really want from life, realize you deserve it, and think positively about your ability to get it. Make your plan, have the inner strength to stick to it, and claim the life you deserve!

THE BEST LIFE
DIET MEAL PLANS

▶ I'm often asked what I eat. It's not that people are wondering if I practice what I preach (I do!) as much as they're looking for good ideas about what to put on their own tables. And it's understandable: even if you're well-versed in nutrition, it's sometimes difficult to translate that information into fresh breakfast, lunch, and dinner options for yourself and, perhaps, for your family, too.

That's where the two meal plans on these next pages come in. They're designed to give you ideas for healthy meals and, if you need it, a more structured way to eat. Some people simply do better on a weight-loss program if their diet is mapped out for them; if you're one of them, these meal plans will work well for you.

The first plan is a week of Oprah's personal menus. You're welcome to follow it if you like—it will definitely give you some great ideas—but it's mainly there to show you how she's adapted the Best Life Diet principles to her own particular needs.

The second plan, two weeks of optimal Best Life menus, is an example of a highly nutritious, highly satisfying way to keep your calorie intake under control. As I mentioned in the chapter about Phase Two, one calorie size does *not* fit all. The basic menu plan is about 1,700 calories, but with some additions (or subtractions) it will cover a wide range of calorie levels: 1,500, 1,600, 1,800, 2,000, and 2,500.

Even if you're eating just 1,500 calories, you'll find the meals surprisingly filling, thanks in part to all of the fiber in this plan. No matter what meals you choose, you'll rack up at least 25 g of fiber.

Here's how to make these meal plans work for you.

▶ Pick a calorie level. If you already know the level at which you can lose weight, stay energized, and not get too hungry, go with that one. Otherwise, it's trial and error. For help on figuring out your calorie level, see my suggestions on page 125.

▶ Check the note under each meal to see if you need more or less food according to your calorie level. If you're on the 1,500-calorie plan, you'll notice you have no daily treat. Add a little more activity to your day and you can move up to activity level 1 or higher and raise your calorie count to a level that does include a treat.

▸ Follow this plan, or mix it up to create your own. The daily plans are just a suggestion; actually, you can choose any breakfast, any lunch, any dinner, any high-calcium snack, and any of the treats, and end the day at the calorie level of your choosing. For instance, you can have Monday's breakfast with Tuesday's lunch, Thursday's dinner, Saturday's snack, and Sunday's treat, and still come out at the daily calorie level of your choice.

▸ Start on any day.

▸ Eat everything: breakfast, lunch, dinner, high-calcium snack, and treat. You need the calories and nutrients to keep your metabolism rolling and to fuel activity.

▸ Make substitutions, if you'd like, but substitute similar foods. For instance, instead of three ounces of lean roast beef, eat three ounces of chicken. Drink one cup of calcium-enriched soymilk (no more than 100 calories) in place of one cup of nonfat milk or have two cups of cauliflower instead of two cups of broccoli.

MEAL PLANS

Oprah's Seven-Day Food Diary

When you read through Oprah's food diary, you'll notice right away that her diet is healthful but far from dull. She averages about 1,700 well-balanced calories daily, and her diet is about 20 percent protein, 30 percent fat (and rich in healthy fats), and 50 percent carbohydrates (good ones like whole grains, fruits, and vegetables). Thanks to all the yogurt and calcium-enriched soymilk she consumes, she's getting an average of about 1,100 mg of calcium daily. Lots of fresh foods prepared simply help keep her sodium levels well within recommended levels. She's a real fiber champion, too, averaging 34 g a day.

DAY 1

Breakfast

Mix for 30 seconds in the blender:

> 4 ounces calcium-enriched orange juice
>
> 1 cup mixed berries
>
> 1 banana
>
> ½ 6-ounce container Yoplait Original Harvest Peach yogurt

Serve with a handful of almonds (about 12)

Snack

2 slices Wasa crispbread topped with:

> 1 tablespoon peanut butter
>
> 1 teaspoon Sarabeth's Kitchen apricot pineapple spreadable fruit

Lunch

1 slice Ezekiel 4:9 Organic Sprouted Whole Grain Bread with
2 teaspoons light mayo, topped with:

> 3 ounces smoked turkey, sliced thin
>
> 1 slice pepper jack cheese
>
> ¼ cup grilled onions brushed with 1 teaspoon olive oil
>
> 1 thin slice avocado
>
> 1 slice tomato
>
> Lettuce

8 ounces sugar-free iced tea

Snack

6 fresh-scooped watermelon balls

Remaining yogurt from breakfast

Dinner

1 cup wild rice with 2 cups mixed vegetables (broccoli, green peas, or carrots) sautéed in 2 teaspoons olive oil

2 skinless, boneless chicken breast cutlets, 6 ounces total, grilled with a little olive oil

DAY 2

Breakfast

¼ cup (dry; about a cup cooked) steel-cut oatmeal topped with:

> 2 tablespoons chopped walnuts

> about ½ cup fresh blueberries

> 1 cup nonfat milk with a splash of hazelnut coffee creamer

Snack

One 6-ounce container Yoplait Light Key Lime Pie yogurt

2 tablespoons chopped almonds for topping

Lunch

2 slices Wasa crispbread topped with:

> 2 ounces turkey

> 1 ounce pepper jack cheese

> 2 fresh basil leaves

1 cup Curried Squash Soup (see recipe on page 209)

Snack

1 pear

1 ounce sharp cheddar cheese

Dinner

Pasta with mixed veggies and chicken: Sauté 1 cup chicken breast strips with 2 cups vegetables in 1 teaspoon olive oil and 1 cup reduced-sodium chicken stock. Add 1 cup cooked Barilla PLUS pasta and the juice of 1 lemon and lots of black pepper.

DAY 3

Breakfast

1 serving Chocolate-Strawberry Smoothie (see recipe on page 198), blended with 1 tablespoon wheat germ

Snack

1 apple, sliced, with 4 teaspoons peanut butter

Lunch

Southwestern Veggie Burger Supreme (see recipe on page 229)

1 orange

8 ounces sugar-free iced tea

Snack

1½ cups vegetables grilled in olive oil

1 hard-boiled egg

Dinner

1 can Slim-Fast Optima Creamy Milk Chocolate

2 slices Wasa crispbread and 1 ounce cheddar cheese

DAY 4

Breakfast

1 slice Ezekiel 4:9 Organic Sprouted Whole Grain Bread toasted, topped with 1 fried egg

2 slices turkey

8 ounces water flavored with ½ of a squeezed lemon

Snack

1 green apple

5 thin Parmesan cheese slices (about 1 ounce)

Lunch

Grilled turkey burger: Ground turkey meat combined with finely chopped green onions, red peppers, and garlic to form a patty, and grilled. Serve on a seven-grain bun and spread with 2 teaspoons reduced-fat mayonnaise and 1 teaspoon mustard.

2 grilled vegetable kabobs composed of cherry tomatoes, mushrooms, zucchini, and onions.

Snack

1 can Slim-Fast Optima French Vanilla

Dinner

Bowl of cherries (about 1 cup) with ½ banana, sliced, and ½ peach, topped with 6-ounce Yoplait Original Harvest Peach yogurt, 3 tablespoons walnuts, and ½ cup Kashi Go Lean cereal.

DAY 5

Breakfast

Best Life Cheerios Mix (see recipe on page 193), topped with ½ cup blueberries and 2 tablespoons almonds, plus 1 cup nonfat milk

Snack

Iced decaf skim latte (12 ounces)

Small handful of cashews (2–3 tablespoons)

Lunch

2 open-faced turkey melts: For each melt, 1 slice Ezekiel 4:9 Organic Sprouted Whole Grain Bread, spread with 1 teaspoon light mayo, topped with 1 ounce turkey, 2 slices tomato, 2 basil leaves, and 1 slice cheddar cheese. Melt in a toaster oven.

Rest of the tomato, sliced

1 cup grapes

Snack

1 ounce dark chocolate

Dinner

Grilled Snapper with Eggplant, Squash, and Potatoes (see recipe on page 241)

1 cup brown rice

DAY 6

Breakfast

One 6-ounce container Yoplait Light Key Lime Pie yogurt mixed with ⅓ cup mango and ⅓ cup blueberries, topped with 2 tablespoons walnuts

Snack

½ whole wheat pita dipped in ⅓ cup hummus

Lunch

Arugula, Grapefruit, and Avocado Salad (see recipe on page 211)

2 ounces fresh mozzarella, stuffed into the remaining ½ pita

Snack

2 slices (2 ounces) turkey breast

1 grilled red pepper

Dinner

Slim-Fast Chocolate Banana Smoothie: Blend until smooth: 1 can of Slim-Fast Optima Creamy Milk Chocolate, 1 ripe banana, and 6 ice cubes

3 tablespoons trail mix

DAY 7

Breakfast

1 serving Strawberry-Orange Smoothie (see recipe on page 199)

1 slice Ezekiel 4:9 Organic Sprouted Whole Grain Bread, toasted, with 1 tablespoon peanut butter

Snack

1 slice Wasa crispbread topped with 1 ounce cheddar cheese

Lunch

Fruit bowl: Combine slices of banana, apple, peach, and mango with one 6-ounce container Yoplait Light Boston Cream Pie yogurt and 3 tablespoons chopped walnuts

Snack

1 ounce dark chocolate

Dinner

3 cups mixed-lettuce salad tossed with 2 teaspoons olive oil and a splash of balsamic vinegar and topped with about 2 ounces grilled shrimp

2 beets, 1 ear roasted corn, 1 sliced tomato, and ½ roasted pepper

1 scoop homemade mango sorbet

Two-Week Best Life Meal Plan

This meal plan is designed for a 1,700-a-day calorie count. However, each day also includes adjustments for 1,500-, 1,600-, 1,800-, 2,000-, and 2,500-calorie levels. If you don't see any specific directions for your calorie count (for instance, "Add another ounce of chocolate to your snack"), then you should adhere to the same guidelines specified for the 1,700-calories-a-day level.

Some other considerations:

The plan doesn't include drinks; I'll leave that to you. Just make sure that your drinks are, for the most part, noncaloric. That means you can have water, seltzer, tea, herbal tea, and coffee. If you want to add sugar to your coffee or tea, remember, it's 16 calories per teaspoon (honey is 21 calories). If you need it, have the occasional diet drink, but better yet, try 0-calorie flavored water such Poland Spring lemon-flavored sparkling water, Hint Essence water, and Metro Mint.

Nonfat (skim) milk is used throughout these meal plans. If you prefer 1 percent, go ahead and have it; just keep in mind that you're adding an extra 19 calories per cup. You can also substitute calcium-enriched soymilk for nonfat milk. Choose brands that are about 100 calories or less per cup.

WEEK ONE

MONDAY, DAY 1

Breakfast

- ▶ Mocha: Add 1 teaspoon chocolate syrup and 1 teaspoon instant coffee to a cup of hot nonfat milk.
- ▶ Pear Muffin (see recipe on page 194; you can make these the night before)
- ▶ 1 large apple

   (2,500 CAL/DAY: Add ¼ cup nonfat milk and another teaspoon chocolate syrup.)

Snack

   2,500 CAL/DAY ONLY: 6 ounces flavored low-fat yogurt—about 150 to 180 calories.

Lunch

- ▶ Salmon with Basil Lean Cuisine Spa Cuisine (wild salmon on a bed of whole wheat orzo with yellow and orange carrots and spinach in a basil sauce)
- ▶ 1 cup each: halved cherry tomatoes and diced cucumbers tossed in 2 teaspoons olive oil, 1 teaspoon fresh basil, and a splash of red wine vinegar
- ▶ 1 orange

   (2,000 CAL/DAY: Add ½ cup frozen microwaved corn.)

   (2,500 CAL/DAY: Add 1 tablespoon grated Parmesan to salad; 1 cup frozen, microwaved corn with 2 teaspoons trans-fat-free margarine.)

High-Calcium Snack

60 calories' worth of whole grain crackers (such as 2 slices Wasa Fiber Rye crispbread) with 1½ ounces reduced-fat cheddar or Swiss cheese

> (1,800, 2,000, AND 2,500 CAL/DAY: Add 60 calories' worth of whole grain crackers such as 3 Wasa Fiber Rye crispbread.)

Dinner

Pasta with Chicken or Shrimp

- ▶ 2 ounces Barilla PLUS penne or other short whole grain pasta (about 1¼ cups cooked)
- ▶ Top with ½ cup tomato-based pasta sauce (store-bought or Pepper and Olive Tomato Sauce, page 248)
- ▶ 3 ounces cooked shrimp or chicken
- ▶ Serve with mixed green salad: Toss 3 cups mixed greens with vinaigrette (½ teaspoon Dijon, 2 teaspoons olive oil, and ½ teaspoon balsamic vinegar)

> (1,500–1,600 CAL/DAY: Have 1½ teaspoons olive oil instead of 2 teaspoons. Pump up the taste with 2–5 sprays of Wish-Bone Salad Spritzer, any flavor.)

> (2,000 CAL/DAY: Have 4 ounces shrimp or chicken and a tablespoon Parmesan cheese.)

> (2,500 CAL/DAY: Have another ½ ounce pasta [about another ½ cup cooked], 4 ounces shrimp or chicken, and a tablespoon Parmesan cheese.)

Treat (anytime during the day)

1 ounce dark chocolate

> (1,500 CAL/DAY: Skip the treat.)

> (1,600 CAL/DAY: .75 ounce)

> (1,800 CAL/DAY: 1.5 ounces)

> (2,000 CAL/DAY: 2 ounces)

> (2,500 CAL/DAY: 2.25 ounces)

TUESDAY, DAY 2

Breakfast

▶ Best Life Kashi Go Lean Mix (see recipe on page 193) topped with 2 tablespoons pecans or other unsalted nut of your choice and 1 cup nonfat milk

▶ ½ grapefruit

(2,500 CAL/DAY: Add another 50 calories of cereal—add more of one of the cereals in the mix, or if you've made it in bulk, add ¼ cup more of the cereal mix.)

Snack

2,500 CAL/DAY ONLY: Iced Vanilla Soy Latte (see recipe on page 272) with 1 graham cracker (preferably whole wheat)

Lunch

▶ Nut Butter and Pear Sandwich: On 2 slices whole wheat bread, spread 2 tablespoons almond or other nut butter of your choice, and add ½ pear, thinly sliced, and 1 teaspoon honey.

▶ ½ cup carrot sticks.

(2,000 CAL/DAY: Add ½ tablespoon nut butter and 1 teaspoon honey.)

(2,500 CAL/DAY: Add 1 tablespoon nut butter and 2 more teaspoons honey; have 1 cup nonfat milk.)

High-Calcium Snack

Maple-Nut Yogurt: Stir 1 teaspoon maple syrup and 1 tablespoon walnut pieces into 6 ounces (¾ cup) low-fat plain yogurt.

(1,800, 2,000, AND 2,500 CAL/DAY: Add another teaspoon maple syrup and another tablespoon walnuts.)

Dinner

▶ Lemon and Herb Grilled Trout (see recipe on page 242)

▶ 5-inch ear of corn, grilled along with the fish

▶ Sautéed Sugar Snap Peas with Ginger (see recipe on page 256)

(1,500–1,600 CAL/DAY: Have ½ ear of the corn.)

(2,000 CAL/DAY: Have 1 large ear of corn [8 inches] instead of a medium ear.)

(2,500 CAL/DAY: Have 1 large ear of corn [8 inches] instead of a medium ear and another serving of Sautéed Sugar Snap Peas with Ginger.)

Treat (anytime during the day)

1 Skinny Cow ice cream cone (150 calories), any flavor

(1,500 CAL/DAY: Skip the treat.)

(1,600 CAL/DAY: 1 Skinny Cow fudge bar, 100 calories)

(1,800 CAL/DAY: Skinny Cow ice cream cone plus a tablespoon of semisweet chocolate chips.)

(2,000 CAL/DAY: Skinny Cow ice cream cone plus 2½ tablespoons semisweet chocolate chips.)

(2,500 CAL/DAY: Skinny Cow ice cream cone plus 3 tablespoons semisweet chocolate chips.)

WEDNESDAY, DAY 3

Breakfast

▶ 1 serving Chocolate-Strawberry Smoothie (see recipe on page 198)

▶ 1½ slices Ezekiel 4:9 Organic Sprouted Whole Grain Bread or other high-fiber (3 g fiber per slice) bread spread with 1 tablespoon peanut or almond butter

(2,500 CAL/DAY: Have 2 slices bread instead of 1½.)

Snack

2,500 CAL/DAY ONLY: Slim-Fast Chocolate Mint Crisp snack bar and ½ cup nonfat or 1 percent milk or calcium-enriched soymilk

Lunch

- ▸ Strawberry-Peach Chicken Salad (see recipe on page 219). Take undressed salad to work; add dressing before eating.

- ▸ 90 calories whole grain crackers (e.g., 3 slices Wasa Fiber Rye crispbread) with 1 ounce reduced-fat cheddar or Swiss cheese

  (2,000 CAL/DAY: Add 60 calories whole grain crackers [e.g., 2 more slices Wasa Fiber Rye crispbread].)

  (2,500 CAL/DAY: Have another portion of Strawberry-Peach Chicken Salad [in other words, you'll eat half the recipe in total]; skip the cheese.)

High-Calcium Snack

- ▸ 12-ounce skim-milk latte
- ▸ 8 almonds

(1,800, 2,000, AND 2,500 CAL/DAY: Add 7 almonds.)

Dinner

- ▸ Steak salad: In a small frying pan, sear a 4-ounce filet mignon steak in 1½ teaspoons hot canola oil for 4 minutes on each side (for medium-rare). Let stand for 10 minutes.

- ▸ Meanwhile, toss 3 cups mixed greens, ⅓ cup white button mushrooms, and 1 tablespoon crumbled blue cheese or Gorgonzola or goat cheese with 1 tablespoon olive oil–based dressing of your choice. Slice the steak and lay the strips on top of the salad.

- ▸ Serve with a baked sweet potato topped with 1 tablespoon low-fat plain yogurt and 1 tablespoon reduced-fat sour cream.

  (1,500–1,600 CAL/DAY: Skip the blue or goat cheese in the salad.)

  (2,000 CAL/DAY: Add ½ tablespoon salad dressing.)

  (2,500 CAL/DAY: Add 1 extra ounce filet mignon, ½ tablespoon dressing, 1 tablespoon blue or goat cheese, and 1–2 tablespoons low-fat yogurt for potato.)

Treat (anytime during the day)

150 calories popcorn, such as Pop Secret 94 Percent Fat Free Butter Popcorn. Depending on the brand, that's about 4–8 cups. Check the label for 0 g trans fat.

>   (**1,500 CAL/DAY**: Skip the treat.)

>   (**1,600 CAL/DAY**: 100 calories popcorn, about 3½–5 cups.)

>   (**1,800 CAL/DAY**: Add 1 tablespoon mixed nuts.)

>   (**2,000 CAL/DAY**: Add 2 tablespoons mixed nuts.)

>   (**2,500 CAL/DAY**: Add 3 tablespoons mixed nuts.)

THURSDAY, DAY 4

Breakfast

▶ Yogurt, fruit, and nuts: Combine 6 ounces 150-to-170-calorie low-fat fruit-flavored yogurt; ¼ cup low-fat plain yogurt; ¾ cup blueberries; ⅓ cup All-Bran; 2 tablespoons walnuts or other unsalted nut of your choice

>   (**2,500 CAL/DAY**: Add 1 tablespoon nuts.)

Snack

>   **2,500 CAL/DAY ONLY**: 1 sliced pear with 1½ ounces reduced-fat cheese

Lunch

▶ Hummus Sandwich: Stuff a medium (120-calorie) whole wheat pita with

>   ⅓ cup hummus

>   1 slice reduced-fat cheese, such as Cabot 50% Light cheddar

>   a few cherry tomatoes, halved

Serve with

>   ½ cup cherry tomatoes

>   ½ cup carrot sticks or baby carrots

▶ ½ grapefruit

(2,000 cal/day: Have a total of ½ cup hummus and add another ½ cup cherry tomatoes.)

(2,500 cal/day: Have ½ cup hummus and add another ½ cup cherry tomatoes, one kiwi, and 4 ounces fruit-flavored yogurt— about 110 calories.)

High-Calcium Snack

Slim-Fast Optima Shake

> (1,800, 2,000, and 2,500 cal/day: Add ½ graham cracker [preferably whole wheat].)

Dinner

▶ Mango and Black Bean Salad with Grilled Chicken (see recipe on page 218)

▶ ¾ ounce baked tortilla chips, about 14, such as Guiltless Gourmet chips

> (1,500–1,600 cal/day: Cut back to ½ ounce chips [about 9].)

> (2,000 cal/day: Add ¼ ounce chips [about 5].)

> (2,500 cal/day: Have ⅓ of the Mango and Black Bean Salad with Grilled Chicken recipe instead of ¼ [as the recipe specifies], along with ¾ ounce chips.)

Treat (anytime during the day)

3 tablespoons chocolate-covered peanuts or almonds or other 150-calorie snack

> (1,500 cal/day: Skip the treat.)

> (1,600 cal/day: 2 tablespoons chocolate-covered nuts or other 100-calorie snack.)

> (1,800 cal/day: ¼ cup chocolate-covered nuts or other 210-calorie snack.)

> (2,000 cal/day: ⅓ cup chocolate-covered nuts or other 280-calorie snack.)

> (2,500 cal/day: ⅓ cup chocolate-covered nuts or other 280-calorie snack, plus ⅓ cup nonfat milk.)

FRIDAY, DAY 5

Breakfast On the Go

- ▶ Fiber One chewy bar
- ▶ 1 cup nonfat or 1 percent milk or calcium-enriched soymilk (grab a carton or put it in your thermos)
- ▶ 1 banana
- ▶ 6 almonds

 (**2,500 CAL/DAY**: Have a total of 14 almonds.)

Snack

 2,500 CAL/DAY ONLY: 6 ounces low-fat fruit yogurt (about 150 to 170 calories).

Lunch, at the Salad Bar

- ▶ 2 cups raw spinach *or* mixed greens
- ▶ ½ cup garbanzo beans *or* any other plain, undressed beans
- ▶ ½ cup chicken breast strips *or* plain tuna *or* tofu
- ▶ 2½ tablespoons reduced-calorie dressing *or* 1½ tablespoons regular oil-based dressing
- ▶ 1 teaspoon bacon bits (optional)
- ▶ 1 slice whole grain bread or a small roll

 (**2,000 CAL/DAY**: Have another ¼ cup garbanzos and add ½ cup shredded carrots.)

 (**2,500 CAL/DAY**: Have another ¼ cup garbanzos; add ½ cup shredded carrots, 1 slice bread, and 1 tablespoon reduced-calorie dressing or ½ tablespoon regular dressing.)

High-Calcium Snack

- ▶ 2 slices Wasa crispbread (such as Multigrain or Fiber Rye) spread with 2 teaspoons jam
- ▶ 1 cup nonfat milk

 (**1,800, 2,000, AND 2,500 CAL/DAY**: Add another slice Wasa crispbread.)

Dinner

Quick and Healthy Microwave Dinner

▶ Lemongrass Chicken Lean Cuisine Spa Cuisine (roasted chicken tenderloins in a lemongrass coconut sauce served over brown rice with broccoli, carrots, baby corn, and yellow carrots)

▶ ½ cup shelled frozen edamame (microwaved along with the Lean Cuisine) tossed with ½ grated carrot, 1 teaspoon fresh cilantro, 1 tablespoon olive oil, and 2 teaspoons balsamic vinegar

(1,500–1,600 CAL/DAY: Cut back to 2 teaspoons olive oil.)

(2,000 CAL/DAY: For dessert, have 1 cup sliced papaya with a spritz of lime juice, or 1 orange.)

(2,500 CAL/DAY: Add an extra ½ cup of edamame to the salad, and for dessert have 1 cup sliced papaya with a spritz of lime juice, or 1 orange.)

Treat (anytime during the day) 1 ounce olive oil potato chips, such as Best Health Olive Oil Cracked Pepper or Rosemary, or Terra chips, or another 150-calorie treat

(1,500 CAL/DAY: Skip the treat.)

(1,600 CAL/DAY: 0.66 ounces chips or another 100-calorie treat.)

(1,800 CAL/DAY: 1.33 ounces chips or another 210-calorie treat.)

(2,000 CAL/DAY: 1.8 ounces chips or another 280-calorie treat.)

(2,500 CAL/DAY: 2 ounces chips or another 300-calorie treat.)

SATURDAY, DAY 6

Breakfast

▶ Spinach and Cheese Omelet (see recipe on page 201)

▶ 1 cup raspberries topped with 6 ounces low-fat vanilla yogurt

(2,500 CAL/DAY: Add 1 slice whole wheat toast.)

Snack

2,500 CAL/DAY ONLY: 1 cup 8th Continent vanilla soymilk with ½ apple spread with 1 teaspoon peanut butter

Lunch

Ham and tomato couscous (you can make this the night before and take it to work in a plastic container). Combine:

▶ 1 cup cooked whole wheat couscous, such as Fantastic Foods or Casbah brands, cooked according to package directions, without any added fat

▶ 2 ounces ham with less than 500 mg sodium per 56 g (2 ounces), such as any of the Healthy Choice hams, Oscar Mayer Lower Sodium ham, or Applegate Farms Uncured Black Forest Ham

▶ ½ cup cherry tomatoes, halved

▶ 1 ounce mozzarella, diced (preferably fresh mozzarella)

▶ 1½ teaspoons olive oil

▶ 1 tablespoon chopped fresh parsley, basil, or other herb of your choice

▶ 1 teaspoon lemon juice or to taste

   (2,000 CAL./DAY: Have another ¼ cup cooked couscous.)

   (2,500 CAL/DAY: Have another ¼ cup cooked couscous and another ½ cup tomatoes, another ½ teaspoon olive oil, and add ½ cup canned no-salt-added garbanzo beans, such as Eden Foods.)

High-Calcium Snack

▶ Mocha Cooler (see recipe on page 271)

   (1,800, 2,000, AND 2,500 CAL/DAY: Add 10 almonds.)

Dinner

▶ Sweet Potato Soup with Yogurt Chive Topping (see recipe on page 208)

▶ Roasted Scallops with Tomato Salsa (see recipe on page 245)

▶ ½ cup cooked brown rice tossed with 1 tablespoon toasted pine nuts

▶ 1 orange

   (1,500–1,600 CAL/DAY: Skip the pine nuts.)

(**2,000 CAL/DAY**: Add ¼ cup rice.)

(**2,500 CAL/DAY**: Add ½ cup rice.)

Treat (anytime during the day)

- ▶ 150 calories sorbet, a heaping ½ cup. Check label for calories.

    (**1,500 CAL/DAY**: Skip the treat.)

    (**1,600 CAL/DAY**: 100 calories sorbet, about ½ cup.)

    (**1,800 CAL/DAY**: 210 calories sorbet, about 1 heaping cup.)

    (**2,000 CAL/DAY**: 210 calories sorbet, about 1 heaping cup, plus 1 large peach or 1¼ cups strawberries, sliced.)

    (**2,500 CAL/DAY**: 230 calories sorbet, about 1¼ cups, and 1 large peach or 1¼ cups strawberries, sliced.)

SUNDAY, DAY 7

Breakfast

- ▶ Hot Cereal with Almonds and Apricots: ½ cup dry (about 1 cup cooked) oatmeal, oat bran, or other whole grain cereal (such as Arrowhead Mills Organic Bits O Barley or Mother's Multigrain Hot Cereal) cooked according to package directions with 6 dried apricot halves and 2 tablespoons wheat germ. Top with 8 almonds or other unsalted nut of your choice.

- ▶ 1 cup nonfat milk

    (**2,500 CAL/DAY**: Start with ⅔ cup dry oatmeal or other cereal instead of ½ cup.)

Snack

2,500 CAL/DAY ONLY: 2 pieces Wasa crispbread with 1½ ounces reduced- fat cheddar (such as Cabot 50% Light) or Swiss cheese.

Lunch

- ▶ Chicken Tabbouleh Pita (see recipe on page 226)
- ▶ Salad: 3 cups of mixed greens tossed with 1 tablespoon olive oil–based salad dressing

▶ 1 orange

(2,000 CAL/DAY: Have 1 more tablespoon salad dressing.)

(2,500 CAL/DAY: Have 1 more tablespoon salad dressing and a
6-ounce fruit yogurt, about 150–170 calories.)

High-Calcium Snack

▶ 90 calories high-fiber cereal of your choice (such as ½ cup
Optimum Slim or Fiber One)

▶ 1 cup nonfat milk

(1,800, 2,000, AND 2,500 CAL/DAY: Have 135 calories cereal.)

Dinner

▶ Spicy Beef Fajitas with Fire-Roasted Salsa Guacamole (see recipe on
page 232)

▶ 1½ cups cauliflower florets, steamed and tossed with 1½ teaspoons
olive oil, 1 teaspoon lime juice, 1–2 teaspoons chopped cilantro,
and a dash of salt

(1,500–1,600 CAL/DAY: Skip the olive oil. Instead, have 2–5 sprays
of a Wish-Bone Salad Spritzer, any flavor.)

(2,000 CAL/DAY: Add 1 more tortilla.)

(2,500 CAL/DAY: Add 1 more tortilla and an extra serving of
guacamole.)

Treat (anytime during the day)

▶ Mini Sundae: ½ cup light vanilla ice cream topped with 1 teaspoon
chocolate syrup and 2 teaspoons peanuts

(1,500 CAL/DAY: Skip the treat.)

(1,600 CAL/DAY: ½ cup light vanilla ice cream.)

(1,800 CAL/DAY: ¾ cup light vanilla ice cream topped with
1 teaspoon chocolate syrup and 2 teaspoons peanuts.)

(2,000 CAL/DAY: 1 cup light vanilla ice cream topped with
2 teaspoons chocolate syrup and 2 teaspoons peanuts.)

(2,500 CAL/DAY: 1 cup light vanilla ice cream topped with
2 teaspoons chocolate syrup and 1 tablespoon peanuts.)

WEEK TWO

MONDAY, DAY 8

Breakfast

- ▸ Best Life Cheerios Mix (see recipe on page 193)
- ▸ Top with 1 cup strawberries (or other fruit of your choice) and 2 tablespoons walnuts or other unsalted nuts
- ▸ 1 cup nonfat milk

  (2,500 CAL/DAY: Add 1 more tablespoon nuts.)

Snack

2,500 CAL/DAY ONLY: 1 cup 8th Continent Light chocolate soymilk with 3 squares plain, cinnamon, or honey graham crackers, preferably whole wheat.

Lunch

- ▸ Cheddar and tomato sandwich:

  Between 2 slices whole wheat bread, place 2 ounces reduced-fat cheddar cheese (such as Cabot 50% Light), 2 slices tomato, and 3 to 5 basil leaves. Slice the rest of the tomato, and serve with 1 cup spinach and ½ cup sliced white button mushrooms tossed with 1 teaspoon olive oil and a dash balsamic vinegar.

- ▸ 1 small apple

  (2,000 CAL/DAY: Add 2 cups spinach and 1 teaspoon olive oil to the salad, and have 1 medium apple.)

  (2,500 CAL/DAY: Add 2 cups spinach, ½ cup garbanzo beans, and 1 teaspoon olive oil to the salad, and have 1 large apple.)

High-Calcium Snack

- ▸ 1 Slim-Fast Optima Shake

  (1,800, 2,000, AND 2,500 CAL/DAY: Add 1 slice Wasa crispbread.)

Dinner

- ▸ Arugula, Grapefruit, and Avocado Salad (see recipe on page 211)

- 4 ounces snapper (or other white fish) broiled and served with a spritz of lemon juice
- 1 cup cooked whole wheat couscous with 1 tablespoon lemon juice and 1 tablespoon chopped parsley

  (1,500–1,600 CAL/DAY: Have ¾ cup couscous.)

  (2,000 CAL/DAY: Have 1½ cups couscous.)

  (2,500 CAL/DAY: Have 6 ounces snapper instead of 4 ounces and an extra ½ cup couscous; toss couscous with 1 teaspoon olive oil.)

Treat (anytime during the day)

- 140- to 160-calorie granola bars (such as Nature Valley Sweet & Salty Nut bars, Nature Valley Chewy Trail Mix bars), or Kashi TLC Chewy bars (all flavors except Cherry Dark Chocolate)

  (1,500 CAL/DAY: Skip the treat.)

  (1,600 CAL/DAY: Have a 100-calorie bar, such as a Quaker Chewy Granola bar.)

  (1,800 CAL/DAY: Have a 200- to 210-calorie bar, such as a Nature Valley Roasted Nut Crunch or Almond Crunch bar.)

  (2,000 CAL/DAY: Have a 200- to 210-calorie bar, such as a Nature Valley Roasted Nut Crunch or Almond Crunch bar, and 1½ tablespoons semisweet chocolate chips.)

  (2,500 CAL/DAY: Have a 200- to 210-calorie bar, such as a Nature Valley Roasted Nut Crunch or Almond Crunch bar, and 2 tablespoons semisweet chocolate chips.)

TUESDAY, DAY 9

Breakfast

- Pumpkin Spice Muffin (see recipe on page 196) spread with 2 teaspoons peanut butter or almond butter
- 1 cup nonfat milk
- 3 strawberries

  (2,500 CAL/DAY: Add 1½ teaspoons peanut butter or almond butter.)

Snack

> **2,500 CAL/DAY ONLY:** 1 cup low-fat plain yogurt with 1 tablespoon Grape Nuts and 1 teaspoon raisins

Lunch

▶ Speedy Southwestern Salad: Combine ¾ cup reduced-sodium or no-salt-added black beans with 1 cup corn kernels, fresh or frozen, and cooked, or no-salt-added canned corn; ½ cup diced red pepper; 3 tablespoons shredded cheddar, jack, or other cheese; and 2 tablespoons salsa.

> **(2,000 CAL/DAY:** Add ¼ cup no-salt-added black beans and 1 tablespoon shredded cheddar to the salad.)

> **(2,500 CAL/DAY:** Add ½ cup no-salt-added black beans; 2 tablespoons shredded cheddar, jack, or other cheese; and 2 teaspoons olive oil to salad.)

High-Calcium Snack

▶ 12-ounce skim latte and ½ unfrosted or undipped biscotti

> **(1,800, 2,000, AND 2,500 CAL/DAY:** Have a whole undipped biscotti.)

Dinner

▶ Spaghetti with Meat Sauce Lean Cuisine (spaghetti served with beef sauce made with tomatoes, sliced mushrooms, and basil)

▶ 2 cups of mixed greens tossed with 1 cup cherry tomatoes, 1 tablespoon toasted pine nuts, 1 tablespoon olive oil, and a splash of balsamic vinegar

> **(1,500–1,600 CAL/DAY:** Have only 2 teaspoons of olive oil.)

> **(2,000 CAL/DAY:** Have a 1-ounce slice of crusty whole grain bread.)

> **(2,500 CAL/DAY:** Have a 1-ounce slice of crusty whole grain bread and add ¼ cup chopped avocado to the salad.)

Treat (anytime during the day)

▶ 1 Skinny Cow ice cream sandwich

(1,500 CAL/DAY: Skip the treat.)

(1,600 CAL/DAY: Skip the ice cream sandwich; have 2 tablespoons bittersweet chocolate chips.)

(1,800 CAL/DAY: 1 Skinny Cow ice cream sandwich plus 2 tablespoons bittersweet chocolate chips.)

(2,000 CAL/DAY: 1 Skinny Cow ice cream sandwich plus 3 tablespoons bittersweet chocolate chips.)

(2,500 CAL/DAY: 1 Skinny Cow ice cream sandwich plus 1 banana and 1 tablespoon bittersweet chocolate chips.)

WEDNESDAY, DAY 10

Breakfast

- ▶ 2 eggs, scrambled with 1 teaspoon olive oil or 2 teaspoons 0 g trans fat margarine, with 1 slice whole wheat toast
- ▶ 1 cup raspberries
- ▶ 1 cup nonfat milk

  (2,500 CAL/DAY: Add ½ more slice toast.)

Snack

  (2,500 CAL/DAY ONLY: ½ cup part-skim ricotta combined with 4 chopped olives and served with 1 slice Wasa crispbread.)

Lunch

- ▶ Turkey and Cheese Sandwich:

  2 slices whole wheat bread spread with 2 teaspoons light mayonnaise (such as Hellmann's Canola Cholesterol Free) and filled with 2 ounces turkey breast, preferably with less than 500 mg sodium per 2 ounces, such as Healthy Choice or Applegate Farm brands; 1 ounce Swiss cheese or other hard cheese; 2 slices tomato

- ▶ The rest of the tomato, sliced, combined with ½ cup cucumber, sliced. Drizzle with 1 teaspoon olive oil and a splash balsamic vinegar.

  (2,000 CAL/DAY: Add 2 ounces turkey breast.)

  (2,500 CAL/DAY: Add 2 ounces turkey breast and 1 apple.)

High-Calcium Snack

Maple-Nut Yogurt: To 6 ounces fat-free plain yogurt, add 1 teaspoon
maple syrup and 1 tablespoon chopped walnuts or other unsalted nuts.

> (1,800, 2,000, AND 2,500 CAL/DAY: Add 2 teaspoons maple
> syrup.)

Dinner

▶ Spinach Salad with Strawberries and Pistachios (see recipe on page
216)

▶ 2 cups lentil or black bean soup, preferably with no more than
500 mg sodium per cup, such as Progresso 99% Fat Free Lentil
soup, or homemade soup (see recipes on pages 205 and 207)

▶ One 5-inch whole wheat pita bread, toasted and broken into pieces
for the soup, if desired

> (1,500–1,600 CAL/DAY: Have 1½ cups lentil soup.)

> (2,000 CAL/DAY: Spread the pita with [or dip it into] 1 teaspoon
> olive oil.)

> (2,500 CAL/DAY: Add 1 more pita and spread with [or dip them
> into] 2 teaspoons olive oil.)

Treat (anytime during the day)

150 calories undipped biscotti (check package label for calorie
counts), plus 1 cup herbal tea

> (1,500 CAL/DAY: Skip the biscotti; have the tea.)

> (1,600 CAL/DAY: 100 calories undipped biscotti, plus 1 cup
> herbal tea.)

> (1,800 CAL/DAY: 210 calories undipped biscotti, plus 1 cup
> herbal tea.)

> (2,000 CAL/DAY: 280 calories undipped biscotti, plus 1 cup
> herbal tea.)

> (2,500 CAL/DAY: 300 calories undipped biscotti, plus 1 cup
> herbal tea.)

THURSDAY, DAY 11

Breakfast

▶ Apple-Cinnamon Oatmeal: Combine ½ cup dry plain oatmeal, cooked to package directions (makes about 1 cup), with 1 small apple, chopped; 2 tablespoons walnuts or other unsalted nut of your choice; 1 teaspoon brown sugar or honey; and a dash cinnamon

▶ 1 cup nonfat milk (you can cook the oatmeal with the milk, if you'd like)

(2,500 CAL/DAY: Add 1 tablespoon walnuts or other unsalted nut of your choice.)

Snack

2,500 CAL/DAY ONLY: Have a low-fat fruit-flavored yogurt (150–170 calories.)

Lunch

▶ Arugula and Tuna Salad with Ricotta Salata (see recipe on page 220)

▶ One 1-ounce slice crusty whole grain bread with 2 tablespoons reduced-fat shredded mozzarella cheese melted on top

▶ 1 fresh peach or ½ cup peaches canned in juice or water

(2,000 CAL/DAY: Add one 1-ounce slice crusty whole grain bread.)

(2,500 CAL/DAY: Add one 1-ounce slice crusty whole grain bread and have 1 peach with ⅓ cup low-fat vanilla yogurt.)

High-Calcium Snack

▶ Smoothie: blend together 1 cup nonfat milk and ½ cup each of unsweetened frozen raspberries and blackberries

(1,800, 2,000, AND 2,500 CAL/DAY: Add ½ banana.)

Dinner

▶ Baked Pasta with Pumpkin and Spinach (see recipe on page 251)

▶ 2 cups mixed greens and ½ cup cherry tomatoes tossed with 120–150 calories of oil-and-vinegar-based dressing (preferably olive oil based)

(**1,500–1,600 cal/day:** Have 100 calories of salad dressing.)

(**2,000 cal/day:** Add ½ cup grapes for dessert.)

(**2,500 cal/day:** Add 1 tablespoon Parmesan cheese to the pasta and have 1 cup grapes for dessert.)

Treat (anytime during the day)

▶ One 4-ounce pudding snack cup (such as Kozy Shack or Jell-O), 140–150 calories

(**1,500 cal/day:** Skip the treat.)

(**1,600 cal/day:** 100 calories pudding [check the package label for calorie counts] or a pudding pop bar.)

(**1,800 cal/day:** Top pudding with 1 tablespoon chopped pecans.)

(**2,000 cal/day:** Top pudding with 2 tablespoons chopped pecans and 8 chocolate chips.)

(**2,500 cal/day:** Top pudding with 2 tablespoons chopped pecans and 12 chocolate chips.)

FRIDAY, DAY 12

Breakfast

▶ Strawberry-Orange Smoothie (see recipe on page 199)

▶ 1½ slices high-fiber (at least 3 g per slice) whole wheat bread, toasted, with 1 tablespoon peanut butter

(**2,500 cal/day:** Add 2 more tablespoons peanut butter.)

Snack

2,500 cal/day only: Dip 5 baked tortilla chips in a layered dip of ¼ cup fat-free refried beans, ¼ cup shredded reduced-fat cheddar or jack cheese, and 2 tablespoons salsa.

Lunch

▶ Chicken, Cashew, and Salad Wrap: Combine 2 cups mixed green salad, tossed, with 2 tablespoons light ranch dressing, ½ grilled skinless, boneless chicken breast, sliced, and 1½ tablespoons cashews. Wrap in a 120- to 130-calorie whole wheat tortilla.

(2,000 CAL/DAY: Add ¼ cup chicken.)

(2,500 CAL/DAY: Add ¼ cup chicken and 1½ tablespoons cashews. Also have 1 orange for dessert.)

High-Calcium Snack

▶ ¾ cup low-fat plain yogurt mixed with 1½ tablespoons raisins (1 miniature box)

(1,800, 2,000, AND 2,500 CAL/DAY: Add 1½ tablespoons more raisins.)

Dinner

▶ 2 Tomato-Basil Mini Pizzas (see recipe on page 253). (Or have 360 calories of a frozen vegetarian pizza with a whole grain crust, such as ⅓ of Amy's Cheese and Pesto Pizza with Whole Wheat Crust or ¼ of DiGiorno Harvest Wheat Roasted Vegetable Pizza.)

▶ 2 cups mixed green salad tossed with 1 chopped scallion, ¼ cup chickpeas, 2 teaspoons olive oil, 1 teaspoon balsamic vinegar, and herbs to taste

(1,500–1,600 CAL/DAY: Skip the chickpeas.)

(2,000 CAL/DAY: Add 1 more teaspoon olive oil.)

(2,500 CAL/DAY: Add 1 more teaspoon olive oil plus another ¼ cup chickpeas.)

Treat (anytime during the day)

▶ ½ cup regular ice cream (140–150 calories), such as Breyers

(1,500 CAL/DAY: Skip the treat.)

(1,600 CAL/DAY: Have ½ cup light ice cream or frozen yogurt, [about 100–110 calories].)

(1,800 CAL/DAY: Have ¾ cup regular ice cream.)

(2,000 CAL/DAY: Have 1 cup regular ice cream.)

(2,500 CAL/DAY: Have 1 cup regular ice cream plus 1 tablespoon chocolate or caramel syrup.)

SATURDAY, DAY 13

Breakfast

▶ 2 Kashi Go Lean whole grain waffles topped with 1 cup low-fat plain yogurt, 2 teaspoons honey, ½ cup sliced strawberries, and 1 tablespoon chopped almonds or other unsalted nut of your choice

(2,500 CAL/DAY: Add 1 more tablespoon chopped almonds or other unsalted nut of your choice.)

Snack

2,500 CAL/DAY ONLY: 1 cup 8th Continent vanilla soymilk and 1 small banana.

Lunch

▶ Tomato, White Bean, and Basil Salad: Combine 1 cup halved grape tomatoes and ½ cup rinsed and drained white beans. Whisk together 1 tablespoon olive oil, 1 tablespoon white balsamic vinegar or rice vinegar, and 1 teaspoon fresh minced basil. Mix with beans and tomatoes.

(2,000 CAL/DAY: Add ⅓ cup white beans and ½ cup grape tomatoes.)

(2,500 CAL/DAY: Add ⅔ cup white beans and ½ cup grape tomatoes.)

High-Calcium Snack

▶ Raspberry Ricotta: Combine ⅓ cup part-skim ricotta cheese with ¼ cup raspberries and 2 teaspoons raspberry jam

(1,800, 2,000, AND 2,500 CAL/DAY: Add another tablespoon ricotta and 1 teaspoon raspberry jam.)

DINNER

▶ Vegetarian Chili (see recipe on page 251), topped with 2 tablespoons reduced-fat shredded cheddar cheese and ¼ cup shredded Monterey jack, served over ½ cup cooked brown rice

(1,500–1,600 CAL/DAY: Have just ¼ cup brown rice.)

(2,000 CAL/DAY: Add ¼ cup brown rice.)

(2,500 CAL/DAY: Add ½ cup brown rice.)

Treat (anytime during the day)

1 ounce dark chocolate

(1,500 CAL/DAY: Skip the treat.)

(1,600 CAL/DAY: .75 ounce dark chocolate.)

(1,800 CAL/DAY: 1.5 ounces dark chocolate.)

(2,000 CAL/DAY: 2 ounces dark chocolate.)

(2,500 CAL/DAY: 2.25 ounces dark chocolate.)

SUNDAY, DAY 14

Breakfast

▶ Salmon and Spinach Frittata (see recipe on page 200)

▶ 1 cup raspberries combined with ½ cup blackberries, fresh or unsweetened frozen

▶ Café au lait made with ¾ cup nonfat milk, ¾ cup coffee, and 1 teaspoon café au lait coffee mix

(2,500 CAL/DAY: Add ½ slice whole wheat bread.)

Snack

(2,500 CAL/DAY ONLY: 1 ounce mozzarella string cheese and 1 large apple.)

Lunch

▶ Kale and White Bean Soup (see recipe on page 204)

▶ 1 whole grain English muffin, toasted and spread with 2 tablespoons hummus

(2,000 CAL/DAY: Add 3 tablespoons hummus.)

(2,500 CAL/DAY: Have 2 slices crusty whole wheat bread in place of the English muffin, plus 3 more tablespoons hummus.)

High-Calcium Snack

▶ 4 whole wheat crackers (about 65 calories' worth) with 1½ ounces reduced-fat cheese, such as Cabot 50% Light

(1,800, 2,000, AND 2,500 CAL/DAY: Add 3 whole wheat crackers.)

Dinner

▶ Overstuffed Baked Potato: Split 1 large baked potato open and top with 1 cup steamed broccoli florets, 1 tablespoon reduced-fat sour cream, ⅔ cup (3 ounces) cooked skinless chicken breast slices, 3 tablespoons feta cheese, ½ sliced green onion, and 1 teaspoon fresh dill (optional)

(1,500–1,600 CAL/DAY: Leave out 1 tablespoon feta and skip the sour cream [substitute 1 tablespoon low-fat plain yogurt, if desired].)

(2,000 CAL/DAY: Add ¼ cup [1 ounce] cooked chicken breast slices.)

(2,500 CAL/DAY: Add ½ cup cooked broccoli florets, another tablespoon sour cream, another ¼ cup chicken breast slices, and another tablespoon feta.)

Treat (anytime during the day)

▶ 150 calories of 0 g trans fat popcorn, such as Pop Secret 94 Percent Fat Free Butter Popcorn (4–8 cups—check package label)

(1,500 CAL/DAY: Skip the treat.)

(1,600 CAL/DAY: 100 calories 0 g trans fat popcorn [3½–5 cups].)

(1,800 CAL/DAY: 150 calories 0 g trans fat popcorn [4–8 cups], plus 1 tablespoon mixed nuts or other nut of your choice.)

(2,000 CAL/DAY: 150 calories 0 g trans fat popcorn [4–8 cups], plus 2 tablespoons mixed nuts or other nut of your choice.)

(2,500 CAL/DAY: 150 calories 0 g trans fat popcorn [4–8 cups], plus 3 tablespoons mixed nuts or other nut of your choice.)

THE BEST LIFE
RECIPES

A NOTE ABOUT SALT AND SODIUM

In an attempt to keep your diet within the recommended daily limit of 2,300 mg sodium, these recipes use reduced-sodium broths, reduced-sodium soy sauce, and, on occasion, no-salt-added canned tomatoes or beans. If you've been eating a high-sodium diet, some recipes may need a little added salt for your taste (though as you work through Phase Three, your tastes will likely change, and you won't feel the need for as much salt).

If you would like more salt, add a pinch at a time once the food is on your plate. Adding salt this way gives you the most sodium bang for your buck. Just a few salt crystals hitting your tongue taste like a lot more salt than when salt is poured into a dish while it's cooking. Each ⅛ teaspoon of salt has 290 mg of sodium, so use it sparingly!

If salt is a suggested item in the recipe, such as "salt and pepper to taste," then the recipe is analyzed without salt. If salt is a mandatory ingredient, as in the ⅛ teaspoon salt called for in the Pumpkin Spice Muffins (page 196), then it's included in the nutrition analysis.

BREAKFAST

Best Life Cereal Mixes

Each of these mixes contains at least 8 g of fiber. To save time (and storage space!), you can make these mixes in bigger quantities and store them in air-tight containers or plastic bags.

Best Life Cheerios Mix

1 serving (about 1½ cups):

Combine ½ cup Cheerios, ⅔ cup of Weetabix Crispy Flakes & Fiber, and ¼ cup All-Bran

To make in bulk, combine 4½ cups Cheerios, 6 cups Weetabix Crispy Flakes & Fiber (the entire 12-ounce box), and 2¼ cups All-Bran

PER SERVING (WITHOUT MILK), ABOUT: Calories: 169, Protein: 6 g, Carbohydrate: 41 g, Dietary Fiber: 11 g, Total Fat: 2 g, Saturated Fat: 1 g, Cholesterol: 0 mg, Calcium: 128 mg, Sodium: 283 mg.

Best Life Kashi Go Lean Mix

1 serving (about 1⅓ cups):

Combine ¾ cup Kashi Go Lean, ⅓ cup Honey Nut Cheerios, and ¼ cup Wheat Chex

To make it in bulk, combine 10⅔ cups Kashi Go Lean (the entire 14.1-ounce box), 4⅔ cups Honey Nut Cheerios, and 3½ cups Wheat Chex

PER SERVING (WITHOUT MILK), ABOUT: Calories: 188, Protein: 13 g, Carbohydrate: 40 g, Dietary Fiber: 10 g, Total Fat: 2 g, Saturated Fat: 0 g, Cholesterol: 0 mg, Calcium: 120 mg, Sodium: 234 mg.

Best Life Post Bran Flakes Mix

1 serving (about 1¼ cups):

> Combine ½ cup Post Bran Flakes, ½ cup Kashi Honey Toasted Oat Heart-to-Heart, and ¼ cup Fiber One

> To make it in bulk, combine 8¼ cups Post Bran Flakes, 8¼ cups Kashi Heart-to-Heart (the entire 12.4-ounce box), and 4 cups Fiber One

PER SERVING (WITHOUT MILK), ABOUT: Calories: 168, Protein: 6 g, Carbohydrate: 45 g, Dietary Fiber: 14 g, Total Fat: 2 g, Saturated Fat: 0 g, Cholesterol: 0 mg, Calcium: 50 mg, Sodium: 269 mg.

Other Breakfasts

An Oprah Original: Fruit and Yogurt Mix

A healthful way to satisfy a sweet tooth.

1 serving:

> One 6-ounce container Yoplait Light Key Lime Pie yogurt

> ⅓ cup chopped mango

> ⅓ cup blueberries

> 2 tablespoons walnut halves

In a medium bowl, mix the yogurt and fruit. Top with the walnuts.

PER SERVING, ABOUT: Calories: 261, Protein: 8 g, Carbohydrate: 37 g, Dietary Fiber: 3 g, Total Fat: 10 g, Saturated Fat: 1 g, Cholesterol: 0 mg, Calcium: 23 mg, Sodium: 87 mg.

Pear Muffins

A combination of maple syrup and fresh and dried fruit give these high-fiber muffins their sweetness.

MAKES 12 MUFFINS

> Nonstick cooking spray

> 1¼ cups nonfat milk

> ⅓ cup maple syrup

¼ cup canola oil

1 egg, lightly beaten

2 cups All-Bran cereal (Original, not Extra Fiber)

¾ cup whole wheat flour

½ cup all-purpose flour

1 tablespoon baking powder

¾ teaspoon ground nutmeg

¼ teaspoon salt

1 large unpeeled pear, shredded (about 1 cup)

½ cup chopped prunes (dried plums) with orange essence

2 tablespoons toasted wheat germ

Preheat the oven to 350 degrees F. and place the rack in the center of the oven. Lightly coat a 12-cup muffin pan with cooking spray.

In a medium bowl, mix the milk, maple syrup, oil, and egg. Stir in the All-Bran and let stand 5 minutes.

In another bowl, whisk together the flours, baking powder, nutmeg, and salt. Make a well in the center of the dry ingredients and pour in the bran mixture. Stir just until the dry ingredients are moistened. Fold in the pear and dried plums.

Divide the batter equally among the prepared muffin cups. Sprinkle ½ teaspoon of wheat germ over each muffin. Bake 20 to 25 minutes, or until the tops of the muffins feel springy when pressed gently. Remove the pan from the oven and allow the muffins to cool in the pan on a wire rack for 10 minutes before removing them from the pan. Serve warm or cool.

PER SERVING, ABOUT: Calories: 184, Protein: 5 g, Carbohydrate: 32 g, Dietary Fiber: 5 g, Total Fat: 6 g, Saturated Fat: 1 g, Cholesterol: 18 mg, Calcium: 155 mg, Sodium: 211 mg.

Pumpkin Spice Muffins

You'd never suspect that these velvety muffins are packed with 8 grams of fiber. Not just for breakfast, they're a real treat for lunch, spread with peanut butter and a little honey.

MAKES 12 MUFFINS

> 2 cups wheat bran
>
> ½ cup boiling water
>
> 1 cup Libby's canned pumpkin
>
> 2 eggs
>
> 1½ cups skim milk
>
> ¼ cup honey
>
> ¼ cup sugar
>
> 3 tablespoons canola oil
>
> 1 cup whole wheat flour
>
> 1 cup all-purpose flour
>
> 1 tablespoon baking soda
>
> 1 tablespoon cinnamon
>
> 1½ teaspoons ginger
>
> ¼ teaspoon clove
>
> ⅛ teaspoon salt
>
> ½ cup chopped walnuts

Preheat the oven to 350 degrees F. and place the rack in the center of the oven. Lightly coat a 12-cup muffin pan with cooking spray.

In a medium mixing bowl, combine bran, water, and pumpkin and let sit for at least 5 minutes.

In another medium mixing bowl, whisk together eggs, milk, honey, sugar, and oil. Combine egg mixture with bran mixture and stir until smooth.

Mix in flours, baking soda, spices, and salt. Stir just until dry ingredients are moistened.

Put a scant ½ cup of batter into each muffin tin. Sprinkle with walnuts and bake for about 20 minutes, until tops are brown and a toothpick tests clean.

Remove the pan from the oven and allow the muffins to cool in the pan on a wire rack for 10 minutes before removing them from the pan. Serve warm or cool.

NOTE: This batter can be kept in the refrigerator for one week and cooked as you need it.

PER MUFFIN, ABOUT: Calories: 257, Protein: 8 g, Carbohydrate: 37 g, Dietary Fiber: 8 g, Total Fat: 12 g, Saturated Fat: 1.3 g, Cholesterol: 36 mg, Calcium: 78 mg, Sodium: 390 mg.

Low-Fat Winter Fruit Granola

The fat content of most commercial granolas is off the charts. Not so this homemade version, which calls for only a small amount of heart-healthy canola oil.

MAKES ABOUT 6 CUPS, OR 24 QUARTER-CUP SERVINGS

> 4 cups regular rolled oats
>
> ¼ cup unprocessed wheat bran
>
> 2 tablespoons canola oil
>
> ⅓ cup maple syrup
>
> 1 teaspoon vanilla extract
>
> ¼ teaspoon almond extract
>
> ½ cup sliced almonds
>
> ½ cup chopped dried pears or apples
>
> ¼ cup dried cranberries
>
> ¼ cup chopped dates
>
> 2 tablespoons chopped crystallized ginger

Preheat the oven to 325 degrees F.

Combine the oats and bran on a large baking sheet.

In a small pan over medium heat, stir in the canola oil, maple syrup, and vanilla and almond extracts. When the mixture begins to bubble, pour it over the oat mixture and mix well.

(*continued*)

Bake for 10 minutes. Add the almonds and stir the mixture thoroughly. Continue to bake until the oats and almonds are lightly toasted, about 10 minutes more, stirring again halfway through.

Stir in the pears or apples, cranberries, dates, and ginger.

Bake until the oats are crisp, about 5 minutes longer.

Remove the pan from the oven and stir the mixture. Let the granola cool for 5 minutes, then stir again.

When completely cool, store the granola in an air-tight container for up to 4 weeks.

PER ¼ CUP, ABOUT: Calories: 108, Protein: 3 g, Carbohydrate: 19 g, Dietary Fiber: 2 g, Total Fat: 3 g, Saturated Fat: 0 g, Cholesterol: 0 mg, Calcium: 19 mg, Sodium: 2 mg.

An Oprah Original: Chocolate-Strawberry Smoothies

This is a delicious way to get soymilk, a good source of vegetarian protein, into your diet.

SERVES 2

> **2 cups 8th Continent Light chocolate soymilk**
>
> **1 medium banana, cut into chunks**
>
> **2 cups (one 10-ounce bag) frozen unsweetened strawberries, such as Cascadian Farm organic**

Place the soymilk, banana, and strawberries in a blender. Cover and blend on high speed for about 1 minute, or until smooth.

Pour into 2 glasses. Serve immediately.

PER SERVING, ABOUT: Calories: 192, Protein: 8 g, Carbohydrate: 38 g, Dietary Fiber: 5 g, Total Fat: 2 g, Saturated Fat: 0 g, Cholesterol: 0 mg, Calcium: 326 mg, Sodium: 183 mg.

Strawberry-Orange Smoothies

These beautiful, deep pink refreshers burst with a day's worth of vitamin C.

SERVES 2

   1½ cups 8th Continent vanilla soymilk

   2 cups (one 10-ounce bag) frozen unsweetened strawberries, partially
      thawed

   1 medium banana, cut into chunks

   ⅓ cup calcium-enriched orange juice

   Honey, to taste, if desired

Place the soymilk, strawberries, banana, and orange juice in a blender.
Cover and blend on high speed for about 1 minute, or until smooth.
Sweeten to taste with honey.

Pour into 2 glasses. Serve immediately.

PER SERVING, ABOUT: Calories: 195, Protein: 6 g, Carbohydrate: 39 g, Dietary
Fiber: 5 g, Total Fat: 3 g, Saturated Fat: 0 g, Cholesterol: 0 mg, Calcium: 308 mg,
Sodium: 131 mg.

Salmon and Spinach Frittata

If possible, use eggs from chickens fed grain spiked with omega-3 fatty acids.
Doing so will give you a full day's worth of omega-3s per serving.

SERVES 4

> ½ tablespoon olive oil
>
> 2 packed cups baby spinach, about 3 ounces
>
> Freshly ground pepper
>
> 5 large eggs, preferably omega-3 eggs
>
> 4–6 ounces salmon, cooked and flaked
>
> ¼ cup crumbled feta cheese
>
> 1 teaspoon chopped fresh dill

Heat the olive oil in a 10-inch nonstick skillet over medium heat. Add the
spinach and cook, stirring frequently, 3 to 4 minutes. Season with pepper
and remove from the heat to cool. Whisk together the eggs, salmon, feta
cheese, dill, and cooked spinach in a bowl.

Preheat the broiler. Pour the mixture back into the skillet, flatten evenly
with a spatula, and cook over medium heat. Lift up the cooked egg around
the edges using a spatula and tilt the skillet to allow uncooked egg to flow
underneath. Cook until the bottom turns golden brown and the egg is
nearly set, about 8 minutes.

Place the skillet under the broiler (if the handle is plastic, wrap it in
aluminum foil or slide the frittata carefully onto a large baking sheet). Broil
until the top of the frittata turns golden brown, 1 to 2 minutes. Slice and
serve.

PER SERVING, ABOUT: Calories: 208, Protein: 17 g, Carbohydrate: 1 g, Dietary
Fiber: 0 g, Total Fat: 14 g, Saturated Fat: 4 g, Cholesterol: 281 mg, Calcium: 101
mg, Sodium: 225 mg.

Spinach and Cheese Omelet

Thanks to the Gruyère, this omelet tastes rich, even without whole eggs. If you don't want to use a fat-free egg product, you can substitute egg whites—though you'll need a lot, about sixteen to twenty.

SERVES 4

> 1 9-ounce box frozen spinach, such as Green Giant
>
> ¼ cup chopped, drained jarred roasted red bell peppers
>
> 2 teaspoons olive oil
>
> Two 8-ounce cartons (2 cups) fat-free egg product, such as Better'n Eggs
>
> ½ cup shredded Gruyère cheese
>
> Coarse-ground black pepper

Microwave the spinach as directed on the box; drain well. Place in a small mixing bowl and stir in roasted peppers. Set aside.

In a 10-inch nonstick skillet, heat 1 teaspoon of the olive oil over medium heat. Pour 1 carton of egg product into skillet; cook 2 to 3 minutes, or until set but still moist on top, lifting edges occasionally to allow uncooked egg product to flow to the bottom of skillet.

Top one side of the cooked egg product with half of the cheese and half of the spinach mixture. With a spatula, loosen the edge of the omelet and fold half of it over the filling. Remove the skillet from the heat; cover it and let it stand for about 1 minute, or until the cheese is melted. Remove the omelet from the skillet.

Repeat with the remaining olive oil, egg product, cheese, and spinach mixture. Sprinkle each omelet with pepper. To serve, cut each omelet in half.

PER SERVING, ABOUT: Calories: 147, Protein: 16 g, Carbohydrate: 5 g, Dietary Fiber: 2 g, Total Fat: 7 g, Saturated Fat: 3 g, Cholesterol: 15 mg, Calcium: 238 mg, Sodium: 286 mg.

SOUP

Italian Vegetable Soup (*Acquacotta*)

Kale is one of those inredibly healthful vegetables (rich in vitamin C, beta-carotene, vitamin B6, and phytonutrients) that we could all do well to eat more of. Here's a perfect way to sneak it in.

SERVES 4

> 1 large bunch kale
>
> 1 tablespoon olive oil
>
> 1 medium onion
>
> 1 large carrot, peeled and chopped
>
> 1 stalk celery, chopped
>
> 2 cloves garlic, minced
>
> 1 cup tomato puree
>
> 2 tablespoons tomato paste
>
> 6 cups water
>
> One 2-inch piece Parmesan cheese rind
>
> Salt and crushed red pepper

Wash the kale well. Remove the leaves from the stems and tear the leaves into medium-size pieces. Set aside.

Place a large nonstick pan over medium-high heat and add the olive oil. Add the onion and cook for about 5 minutes, until softened. Add the carrot, celery, and garlic, and cook for 5 minutes longer, stirring often.

Stir in the tomato puree, tomato paste, and the water. Bring to a boil. Add the Parmesan rind and kale. Reduce the heat and simmer for 30 minutes. Remove the Parmesan rind. Season the soup with salt and red pepper flakes.

PER SERVING, ABOUT: Calories: 127, Protein: 6 g, Carbohydrate: 16 g, Dietary Fiber: 3 g, Total Fat: 6 g, Saturated Fat: 2 g, Cholesterol: 6 mg, Calcium: 162 mg, Sodium: 175 mg.

Mexican Tortilla Soup with Roasted Chicken

This soup's lightly spicy broth is delicious, but the fun is in the fixings: avocado, shredded cheese, and tortilla chips sprinkled on top.

SERVES 4

> 2 tablespoons olive oil
>
> ½ yellow onion, sliced thin
>
> 4 cloves garlic, chopped fine
>
> ¼ teaspoon ground cumin
>
> Salt and freshly ground pepper
>
> 4 cups reduced-sodium chicken broth, such as Health Valley fat-free chicken broth or Pacific Foods low-sodium chicken broth
>
> ½ small roasted chicken, skin and bones discarded, meat shredded
>
> One 14½-ounce can Muir Glen organic Fire Roasted Diced Tomatoes*
>
> 2 tablespoons fresh lime juice
>
> ¼ cup chopped fresh cilantro
>
> 6 small (6-inch) corn tortillas, cut in half, then into ¼-inch strips
>
> ½ ripe avocado, cubed
>
> ¼ cup shredded low-fat Monterey Jack cheese

In a large stockpot over a medium-low flame, heat 1 tablespoon of the olive oil. Add the onions and sauté them until they are soft, about 10 minutes. Add the garlic, cumin, salt, and pepper, and sauté the mixture another minute.

Add the chicken broth, raise the flame to high, and bring to a simmer. Add the shredded chicken, tomatoes, lime juice, and cilantro. Season with salt and freshly ground pepper. Remove the stockpot from the heat and cover.

Meanwhile, in a small skillet over a medium flame, heat the remaining tablespoon of olive oil. Add the tortilla strips and allow them to brown, stirring occasionally, about 5 minutes. Sprinkle them with salt.

To serve, ladle soup into bowls, top with cubed avocado, shredded cheese, and a handful of tortilla strips.

* If fire-roasted tomatoes are unavailable, use regular diced tomatoes.

PER SERVING, ABOUT: Calories: 264, Protein: 11 g, Carbohydrate: 23 g, Dietary Fiber: 4 g, Total Fat: 14 g, Saturated Fat: 3 g, Cholesterol: 21 mg, Calcium: 135 mg, Sodium: 398 mg.

Kale and White Bean Soup

Hearty, healthy soups can be laborious—but not this one. It calls for canned beans, which lops a couple of hours off of the prep time.

SERVES 4

> 1 small bunch kale
>
> 2 teaspoons olive oil
>
> 1 large onion, thinly sliced
>
> 4 cloves garlic, finely chopped
>
> ¼ teaspoon red pepper flakes
>
> One 15-ounce can cannellini beans, drained and rinsed
>
> 3 cups fat-free chicken broth, such as Health Valley fat-free chicken broth or Pacific Foods low-sodium chicken broth
>
> 2 cups water
>
> ½ teaspoon dried oregano
>
> Salt and freshly ground pepper
>
> 2 tablespoons freshly grated Parmesan cheese

Wash the kale well. Remove the leaves from the stems and discard center ribs, and slice the leaves into thin ribbons. Set aside.

Heat the olive oil in a heavy stockpot over a medium-low flame and sauté the onion, stirring occasionally, until it begins to caramelize, about 15 minutes. Add the garlic and red pepper flakes and sauté the mixture another minute.

Add the beans, broth, water, and oregano, and bring to a simmer.

Add the kale and simmer, uncovered, stirring occasionally, until it is tender, about 15 minutes. Season with salt and pepper. Divide the soup among four bowls and sprinkle each serving with equal amounts of Parmesan cheese.

PER SERVING, ABOUT: Calories: 150, Protein: 8 g, Carbohydrate: 21 g, Dietary Fiber: 5 g, Total Fat: 4 g, Saturated Fat: 1 g, Cholesterol: 2 mg, Calcium: 103 mg, Sodium: 157 mg.

Lentil Soup with Turkey Bacon, Peppers, and Herbs

With 18 g of fiber per serving, this soup helps bring you up to the day's fiber recommendation (25 g for women and 38 g for men).

SERVES 6

- 1 tablespoon olive oil
- 1 cup chopped onion
- ⅔ cup chopped carrot
- 1 bell pepper, chopped
- 4 cloves garlic, finely minced
- 3 slices turkey bacon, chopped
- 1½ cups dried lentils
- 5–6 cups fat-free chicken broth, such as Health Valley fat-free chicken broth or Pacific Foods low-sodium chicken broth
- One 14½-ounce can crushed tomatoes
- 3 sage leaves, finely chopped
- 2 large fresh thyme sprigs, finely chopped
- 1 rosemary sprig, finely chopped
- Salt and pepper to taste
- 2 tablespoons chopped fresh cilantro (parsley may be substituted)

In a heavy-bottomed pot over a medium flame, heat the olive oil and sauté the onion, carrot, bell pepper, garlic, and bacon until the vegetables are tender, 5 to 7 minutes.

Stir in the lentils. Add 5 cups chicken broth, tomatoes, sage, thyme, and rosemary; turn up the flame to high and bring the mixture to a simmer. Lower the flame to medium-low and simmer the mixture, uncovered, until the lentils are tender, stirring occasionally, about 45 minutes. Remove the pot from the heat and allow it to cool slightly, about 10 minutes.

Transfer 4 cups of the soup to a food processor or blender. Puree on low speed until smooth. Return the soup to the pot.

To serve, bring the soup back to a simmer, thinning it by adding more broth, if necessary. Season with salt and pepper and sprinkle with chopped cilantro.

Timesaver: Heat 1 teaspoon olive oil in a heavy-bottomed pot over a medium flame. Sauté the turkey bacon then add two 19-ounce cans of Progresso 99% Fat Free Lentil soup and the canned tomatoes. (You don't need the other recipe ingredients.) Simmer for 10 minutes.

PER SERVING, ABOUT: Calories: 255, Protein: 17 g, Carbohydrate: 40 g, Dietary Fiber: 18 g, Total Fat: 4 g, Saturated Fat: 1 g, Cholesterol: 4 mg, Calcium: 73 mg, Sodium: 283 mg.

Tuscan Minestrone Soup

This classic calls for a classic topping: a sprinkle of Parmesan cheese. But if you want to reduce the soup's already low calorie count even more, leave off the cheese—the soup will still taste rich and satisfying.

SERVES 6

> 2 tablespoons olive oil
>
> 1 medium zucchini, cut into ½-inch slices, about 2 cups
>
> 1 medium summer squash, cut into ½-inch slices, about 2 cups
>
> 1 large carrot, finely diced, about ¾ cup
>
> 1 small onion, finely diced, about ¾ cup
>
> 2 cloves garlic, minced
>
> 1 teaspoon Italian seasoning
>
> 4 cups all-natural reduced-sodium chicken broth, such as Health Valley fat-free chicken broth or Pacific Foods low-sodium chicken broth
>
> One 15-ounce can diced tomatoes
>
> One 15-ounce can cannellini beans, drained and rinsed
>
> ½ cup whole wheat Barilla PLUS or elbow pasta
>
> 3 fresh thyme sprigs
>
> Salt and freshly ground pepper
>
> ⅓ cup grated Parmesan cheese
>
> ⅓ cup loosely packed fresh basil, cut into strips

Heat the oil in a Dutch oven over medium-high heat. Add the zucchini, summer squash, carrot, onion, garlic, and Italian seasoning to the Dutch oven and cook, stirring frequently, until the vegetables start to soften, about 10 minutes. Stir in the broth and diced tomatoes, cover the mixture, and bring it to a boil. Add the beans, pasta, and thyme, and cook, uncovered, at a low boil until the pasta is done, about 10 minutes. Remove the thyme sprigs, and season the mixture with salt and pepper. Serve in individual bowls and top each serving with the Parmesan cheese and basil.

PER SERVING, ABOUT: Calories: 193, Protein: 10 g, Carbohydrate: 25 g, Dietary Fiber: 6 g, Total Fat: 7 g, Saturated Fat: 2 g, Cholesterol: 5 mg, Calcium: 130 mg, Sodium: 516 mg.

Carrot and Leek Lentil Soup

The secret to this soup's smooth, smoky flavor is lean turkey bacon, chopped and stirred in at the last minute.

SERVES 8

> 1 tablespoon olive oil
>
> 1 leek, white part only, sliced into thin rounds
>
> 2 large carrots, peeled and cut into ⅛-inch-thick half-moons
>
> 2 garlic cloves, minced
>
> 4 cups all-natural reduced-sodium chicken broth, such as Health Valley fat-free chicken broth or Pacific Foods low-sodium chicken broth
>
> 3 cups water
>
> 1-pound bag dried lentils (about 2⅓ cups), rinsed
>
> One 8-ounce can diced tomatoes
>
> 1 bay leaf
>
> 1 teaspoon chopped fresh thyme
>
> ⅛ teaspoon black pepper
>
> 6 slices turkey bacon, cooked and chopped
>
> ½ cup grated Parmesan cheese, if desired

Heat the olive oil in a Dutch oven or large saucepan over medium-high heat. Add the leek and carrots and cook, stirring frequently, until soft, about 5 minutes. Stir in the garlic and cook for an additional minute. Add the broth, water, lentils, diced tomatoes, bay leaf, thyme, and black pepper, and stir to combine. Cover the pot and bring to a boil. Reduce the heat and simmer, with the lid loose to allow for venting, until the lentils are tender, 35 to 40 minutes. Discard the bay leaf and stir in the bacon. Serve the soup in individual bowls and top with Parmesan cheese.

PER SERVING, ABOUT: Calories: 266, Protein: 19 g, Carbohydrate: 38 g, Dietary Fiber: 18 g, Total Fat: 5 g, Saturated Fat: 1 g, Cholesterol: 8 mg, Calcium: 51 mg, Sodium: 321 mg.

Sweet Potato Soup with Yogurt Chive Topping

Naturally sweet and bursting with beta-carotene (sweet potatoes are a great source of this antioxidant), this soup makes a great first course.

SERVES 4

> 2 teaspoons olive oil
>
> 1 small onion, finely chopped
>
> 1 teaspoon ground cumin
>
> 1 sweet potato, peeled and cubed
>
> 2 cups fat-free chicken broth, such as Health Valley fat-free chicken broth or Pacific Foods low-sodium chicken broth
>
> Salt and freshly ground black pepper
>
> ½ cup nonfat plain yogurt
>
> 3 teaspoons chopped chives

In a heavy-bottomed stockpot over a medium flame, heat the olive oil. Add the onion and cumin and sauté for 10 minutes, stirring frequently. Add the sweet potato and the chicken broth, raise the flame to high, and bring the mixture to a boil. Reduce the heat and simmer the soup until the potato is tender, 25 to 30 minutes. Remove the pot from the heat and allow the soup to cool slightly, about 10 minutes.

Transfer the soup to a food processor or blender. If using a blender, work in batches and do not fill the blender more than half way. Puree the soup at a low speed, until smooth.

Return the soup to the pot, and reheat it. Season the soup with salt and pepper. Whisk in the yogurt and serve with a sprinkling of chives.

PER SERVING, ABOUT: Calories: 80, Protein: 3 g, Carbohydrate: 11 g, Dietary Fiber: 1 g, Total Fat: 2 g, Saturated Fat: 0 g, Cholesterol: 1 mg, Calcium: 81 mg, Sodium: 94 mg.

Curried Squash Soup

You may be surprised to find half-and-half in this recipe, but it's used sparingly. There's just enough added to give the soup a velvety finish. Divided among five servings, the fat is fairly negligible.

SERVES 5

    1 tablespoon olive oil

    1 medium onion, chopped

    1 clove garlic, finely chopped

    1¾ cups reduced-sodium chicken broth or vegetable broth, such as Health Valley fat-free chicken broth, Pacific Foods low-sodium chicken broth, or Health Valley fat-free vegetable broth

    ¼ cup apple juice

    Two 10-ounce boxes frozen winter squash, such as Cascadian Farm organic winter squash, thawed

    2 teaspoons curry powder

    ½ teaspoon coarse salt (kosher or sea salt)

    ¼ cup half-and-half

In a 4-quart saucepan, heat the olive oil over medium heat. Cook the onion and garlic in the oil for 3 to 5 minutes, stirring frequently, until tender.

Stir in the broth, apple juice, squash, curry powder, and salt. Heat the mixture until it boils, stirring occasionally. Simmer, uncovered, for 5 minutes, stirring occasionally. Stir in the half-and-half. Cook for 3 to 5 minutes, stirring occasionally, until hot (do not boil). Serve in individual bowls.

PER SERVING, ABOUT: Calories: 105, Protein: 2 g, Carbohydrate: 15 g, Dietary Fiber: 2 g, Total Fat: 4 g, Saturated Fat: 1 g, Cholesterol: 5 mg, Calcium: 41 mg, Sodium: 231 mg.

Corn Chowder with Shrimp

This soup is a real comfort food, and hearty enough to build a meal around.

SERVES 6

> One 10-ounce box Green Giant frozen Niblets corn in butter sauce
>
> 1 tablespoon olive oil
>
> 1 medium onion, chopped (½ cup)
>
> 1 medium red or green bell pepper, chopped (1 cup)
>
> 1 stalk celery, chopped (⅓ cup)
>
> 2 cloves garlic, finely chopped
>
> 1 cup reduced-sodium chicken broth
>
> 1 large potato, peeled and cut into ½-inch cubes
>
> ½ teaspoon chopped fresh or ¼ teaspoon dried thyme leaves
>
> ⅛ teaspoon cayenne pepper
>
> 2 cups nonfat (skim) milk
>
> 2 tablespoons all-purpose flour
>
> 12 ounces peeled and deveined shrimp, tails removed

Let the frozen corn stand at room temperature to thaw slightly.

In a 4-quart saucepan, heat the olive oil over medium heat. Cook the onion, bell pepper, celery, and garlic in the oil, stirring frequently, until tender. Add the broth, potato, thyme, and cayenne pepper. Heat the mixture until it boils. Reduce the heat; cover and simmer for 10 minutes.

Remove the frozen corn from its pouch; add the corn to the mixture in the saucepan. Heat the soup until it boils, stirring frequently to break up the frozen corn. Pour the milk into a medium bowl; whisk in the flour until smooth. Stir the milk and flour into the mixture in the saucepan. Heat the soup until it boils. Reduce the heat; simmer uncovered about 5 minutes, or until the vegetables are tender and the soup is thickened. Stir in the shrimp; cook for 1 to 2 minutes or until hot. Serve immediately.

PER SERVING, ABOUT: Calories: 242, Protein: 21 g, Carbohydrate: 29 g, Dietary Fiber: 3 g, Total Fat: 4 g, Saturated Fat: 1 g, Cholesterol: 115 mg, Calcium: 159 mg, Sodium: 299 mg.

SALADS

Side Salads

Arugula, Grapefruit, and Avocado Salad

This salad gets a double hit of citrus flavor: the grapefruit segments adorn the greens, while their juice gets mixed into the dressing.

Serves 4

> 2 Ruby Red grapefruits
> 2 tablespoons olive oil
> ¾ teaspoon kosher or sea salt
> 1 avocado, peeled, cored, and diced
> ¼ cup red onion, very thinly sliced (about ½ small red onion)
> 6 cups fresh arugula, rinsed well and patted dry

Remove the skin and pith from the grapefruits. Cut the grapefruits into segments by cutting between and removing the membranes. (Hold fruit over a bowl to catch the juice.) Reserve the juice. Refrigerate the segments until ready to serve.

Place ⅓ cup of the reserved grapefruit juice in a medium mixing bowl. Whisk in the olive oil and salt. Set the mixture aside. Add the avocado and the onion to the dressing. Stir gently.

To serve, place the arugula in a very large bowl. With a slotted spoon, remove the avocado and onion from the dressing and gently toss them with the arugula; there should be just enough dressing to coat the leaves lightly. Place the salad on a platter and garnish it with the grapefruit segments. Drizzle the salad with a little more dressing, if needed.

PER SERVING, ABOUT: Calories: 203, Protein: 3 g, Carbohydrate: 20 g, Dietary Fiber: 6 g, Total Fat: 15 g, Saturated Fat: 2 g, Cholesterol: 0 mg, Calcium: 83 mg, Sodium: 372 mg.

Fennel and Orange Salad

Oranges and cranberries add a healthy dose of vitamin C to this dish and give it a fresh, bright color.

SERVES 6

> 4 navel oranges
>
> ¼ cup sweetened dried cranberries, such as Craisins
>
> 1 head (bulb) fennel
>
> 1 tablespoon extra-virgin olive oil
>
> 1 teaspoon kosher or sea salt
>
> Salt
>
> ¼ cup slivered almonds, toasted and cooled

Peel and segment the oranges, reserving ½ cup of orange juice. (Hold the fruit over a bowl as you separate the segments to catch the juice.) In a small bowl, combine the orange juice and dried cranberries and set aside for 10 minutes so the cranberries can plump.

Clean, trim, and remove any brown or bruised areas of the fennel. Cut the fronds off and reserve. Shave the fennel crosswise using the finest slicing blade on the food processor or mandoline. In a large bowl, toss the shaved fennel with the orange segments, olive oil, and salt. Mince 1 tablespoon of the green fennel fronds and toss them into the salad. Add the plumped cranberries and orange juice to the salad and gently toss it to combine. Cover and chill the salad for at least 30 minutes before serving so the flavors can develop. Season with salt, if desired.

Serve the salad cold and garnish with the toasted almonds and some of the fennel fronds.

PER SERVING, ABOUT: Calories: 120, Protein: 2 g, Carbohydrate: 20 g, Dietary Fiber: 4 g, Total Fat: 5 g, Saturated Fat: 1 g, Cholesterol: 0 mg, Calcium: 71 mg, Sodium: 342 mg.

Spinach and Bacon Salad with Mango and Jicama

Mango and jicama give this classic dish a tropical twist.

SERVES 4

Mango Dressing

⅓ cup mango nectar

3 tablespoons freshly squeezed lime juice

1 teaspoon grated lime zest

2 teaspoons maple syrup

1 tablespoon extra-virgin olive oil

Salt

Salad

4 slices turkey bacon, chopped

2 mangoes

1 small jicama (1 cup of chopped celery may be substituted)

6 ounces baby spinach, washed well

¾ cup sliced white button mushrooms

¼ cup diced red onion

Chopped cilantro

To make the dressing, whisk the mango nectar, lime juice, lime zest, maple syrup, and olive oil in a small bowl. Season with salt.

In a small nonstick skillet set over a medium flame, fry the bacon, stirring often, until crisp. Drain it on paper towels and set aside.

With a small, sharp knife, peel the mangoes. One at a time, set the fruit on one of its narrow edges on a cutting surface and cut ⅛-inch-thick slices off each side until you reach the pit. Cut the remaining fruit from the pit and reserve for another use.

Peel the jicama. Lay it on a cutting surface, flattest side down, and cut it into ½-inch ovals.

In a large bowl, combine the spinach, mushrooms, red onion, and cooked bacon. Drizzle about half of the dressing over the mixture and toss to coat.

Divide the salad equally among four salad plates. Alternate some of the mango and jicama slices over each salad. Drizzle the remaining dressing over the salads and sprinkle each one with chopped cilantro.

PER SERVING, ABOUT: Calories: 240, Protein: 6 g, Carbohydrate: 42 g, Dietary Fiber: 11 g, Total Fat: 7 g, Saturated Fat: 1 g, Cholesterol: 11 mg, Calcium: 81 mg, Sodium: 295 mg.

Radicchio and Spinach Salad with Grapes, Walnuts, and Blue Cheese

Walnut oil, used to make the dressing, is particularly rich-tasting—a little of it goes a long way.

SERVES 3

Walnut-Balsamic Vinaigrette

2 tablespoons walnut oil

3 tablespoons balsamic vinegar

2 teaspoons honey

Salt and freshly ground pepper

Salad

2½ cups chopped radicchio

2½ cups baby spinach, washed well

1 cup seedless red grape halves

¾ cup thinly sliced celery

3 tablespoons walnut pieces

3 tablespoons crumbled blue cheese

To make the dressing, in a small bowl whisk the walnut oil, vinegar, and honey to blend completely. Season the mixture with salt and pepper and set aside.

In a large bowl, combine the radicchio, spinach, grape halves, celery, and walnuts. Toss the salad to combine. Add the blue cheese and vinaigrette and toss to coat.

PER SERVING, ABOUT: Calories: 238, Protein: 5 g, Carbohydrate: 18 g, Dietary Fiber: 2 g, Total Fat: 17 g, Saturated Fat: 3 g, Cholesterol: 6 mg, Calcium: 99 mg, Sodium: 167 mg.

Beet Salad with Baby Greens and Hazelnuts

Cooked beets are one of the easiest vegetables to peel. Once they're roasted, the skins slip right off.

SERVES 4

> **4 red beets**
>
> **¼ cup hazelnuts**
>
> **2 tablespoons red wine vinegar**
>
> **¼ cup extra-virgin olive oil**
>
> **Salt and freshly ground pepper**
>
> **6 cups fresh baby greens, such as spinach or baby mesclun, washed well**
>
> **1 tablespoon Italian parsley, finely chopped**

Preheat the oven to 350 degrees F. Remove and discard the beet greens from the beets. Wrap each beet loosely in foil. Roast the beets for about 1 hour, until they are barely soft to the touch. When they are cool enough to handle, remove the skins and slice the beets into 8 wedges each. Set them aside, covered.

Place the hazelnuts on a pie plate. Place in the oven and toast until they just begin to color and the skins begin to separate, about 5 minutes. When the hazelnuts are cool enough to handle, rub the skins off and squeeze the nuts until they split.

To make the dressing, in a small bowl combine the vinegar, olive oil, salt, and pepper.

Just before serving, divide the dressing in half and, in one bowl, toss the sliced beets and hazelnuts with half of the dressing. In another bowl, toss the greens with the other half of the dressing.

To assemble the salad, arrange a fourth of the greens in the center of each salad plate. Place a fourth of the beets and hazelnuts around the greens. Top with a generous pinch of chopped parsley.

PER SERVING, ABOUT: Calories: 221, Protein: 4 g, Carbohydrate: 11 g, Dietary Fiber: 4 g, Total Fat: 19 g, Saturated Fat: 2 g, Cholesterol: 0 mg, Calcium: 69 mg, Sodium: 101 mg.

Spinach Salad with Strawberries and Pistachios

If strawberries aren't in season, substitute sliced apples or pears.

SERVES 4

Vinaigrette

3 tablespoons extra-virgin olive oil

2 tablespoons balsamic vinegar

1 tablespoon minced red onion

1 teaspoon Dijon mustard

1 teaspoon maple syrup

Salt and freshly ground pepper

Salad

One 6-ounce bag baby spinach, washed well

1 cup thinly sliced strawberries

¼ cup shredded Parmesan cheese

¼ cup coarsely chopped pistachio nuts, toasted and cooled

To make the dressing, whisk together the olive oil, vinegar, red onion, mustard, maple syrup, and salt and pepper to taste, until well combined.

Divide the spinach among four chilled bowls. Top each serving evenly with the strawberries, Parmesan cheese, and pistachio nuts. Drizzle on the dressing and serve.

PER SERVING, ABOUT: Calories: 189, Protein: 5 g, Carbohydrate: 8 g, Dietary Fiber: 3 g, Total Fat: 15 g, Saturated Fat: 3 g, Cholesterol: 4 mg, Calcium: 122 mg, Sodium: 150 mg.

Main Dish Salads

Tarragon Chicken Salad

Serve this salad on a bed of lettuce, or for a heartier meal, use it as a sandwich filling.

SERVES 4

¼ cup slivered almonds

1 teaspoon canola oil

2 boneless, skinless chicken breasts, about 1 pound, or 2 cups of white-meat chicken pieces without skin from a cooked rotisserie chicken

Salt and freshly ground white pepper

½ cup water

¾ cup diced celery (about 2 large stalks)

½ cup sliced white button mushrooms

2 tablespoons fresh French tarragon, minced, plus additional sprigs for garnish, or 2 teaspoons dried tarragon

3 tablespoons nonfat plain yogurt, strained

3 tablespoons light mayonnaise (no more than 50 calories and 5 g fat per tablespoon), such as Hellmann's Canola Cholesterol Free

Heat an 8-inch nonstick sauté pan over medium heat. Toast the almonds until fragrant and just starting to brown. Transfer the almonds to a plate to cool and crisp. If using chicken breasts, increase the heat to medium-high and add the canola oil. Season the chicken on both sides with salt and freshly ground white pepper. When the canola oil is heated, swirl it to cover the bottom of pan. Add the chicken breasts and sear them until lightly browned. Turn the chicken and lightly brown it on the other side. Add the water to the pan, cover, and reduce the heat to medium. Cook the chicken, covered, for 20 minutes, or until breasts are cooked through. Remove the chicken from the pan to cool.

Place the celery in a large mixing bowl with the mushrooms, and add the tarragon. Add the yogurt, mayonnaise, and cooled almonds, and toss the mixture.

When the chicken has cooled, cut it into ½-inch pieces and add them to the dressing, or add the precooked chicken. Gently toss the chicken and salad together and taste. Season the salad with salt and freshly ground white pepper to taste.

Cover and chill until time to serve. Garnish with sprigs of fresh tarragon, if desired.

PER SERVING, ABOUT: Calories: 225, Protein: 29 g, Carbohydrate: 4 g, Dietary Fiber: 1 g, Total Fat: 10 g, Saturated Fat: 1 g, Cholesterol: 66 mg, Calcium: 75 mg, Sodium: 191 mg.

Mango and Black Bean Salad with Grilled Chicken

This dish can be as spicy as you like. Just vary the amount of jalapeño to determine the heat.

SERVES 4

> ½ cup prepared vinaigrette salad dressing, preferably olive oil–based, such as Newman's Own olive oil and vinegar salad dressing
>
> ¼ cup chopped fresh cilantro
>
> 1½ teaspoons grated lime peel
>
> Four 5-ounce boneless, skinless chicken breasts
>
> One 15-ounce can black beans, preferably with no salt added, such as Eden Foods, or reduced sodium, such as Goya low-sodium black beans
>
> ¼ cup chopped red onion
>
> 1–2 jalapeño peppers, seeded and finely chopped
>
> 2 small or 1 large ripe mango
>
> Mixed salad greens, about 8 cups

In a small bowl, combine the salad dressing, cilantro, and lime peel.

In a resealable food-storage bag, place ¼ cup of the dressing and all four of the chicken breasts. Refrigerate for 30 minutes.

Meanwhile, in a medium bowl, combine the black beans, onion, and jalapeño with the remaining dressing and set the mixture aside.

On a cutting board, hold one of the mangoes with one of the narrower sides facing up. Starting ¼ inch from the stem, slice along each side of the pit to cut off the "cheeks." Cut the flesh in a crisscross pattern, taking care not to cut through the skin. Press the skin to turn mango inside out so fruit pops outward. With a spoon or knife, remove the mango cubes. Peel the center section of the mango, then cut off the remaining fruit and chop. Repeat with the remaining mango.

Remove the chicken from the marinade. Discard the marinade. Grill or broil the chicken until it is cooked through. Toss the mango into the bean mixture. Place the greens on a platter. Spoon the black bean salad on top. Slice the chicken and arrange over salad.

PER SERVING, ABOUT: Calories: 461, Protein: 41 g, Carbohydrate: 33 g, Dietary Fiber: 10 g, Total Fat: 18 g, Saturated Fat: 3 g, Cholesterol: 82 mg, Calcium: 123 mg, Sodium: 383 mg.

Strawberry-Peach Chicken Salad

Using yogurt instead of oil makes for a refreshing low-fat salad dressing.

SERVES 4

Strawberry Yogurt Dressing
Two 6-ounce containers Yoplait Original Strawberry yogurt

1 cup sliced fresh strawberries

2 tablespoons red wine vinegar

Salad
6 cups Bibb lettuce leaves or mixed salad greens

1 pound boneless, skinless chicken breasts, cooked and cut into strips

1 cup sliced fresh strawberries

1 medium peach, peeled, pitted, and sliced

2 medium green onions, sliced

Place the dressing ingredients in a blender or food processor. Cover and blend on high speed for about 15 seconds, or until smooth.

Arrange the salad ingredients on four serving plates.

Drizzle with the dressing. Cover and refrigerate any remaining dressing.

PER SERVING, ABOUT: Calories: 274, Protein: 30 g, Carbohydrate: 28 g, Dietary Fiber: 3 g, Total Fat: 5 g, Saturated Fat: 2 g, Cholesterol: 74 mg, Calcium: 211 mg, Sodium: 114 mg.

Arugula and Tuna Salad with Ricotta Salata

This tuna salad is simple to make and incredibly flavorful. You won't miss the traditional mayonnaise-laden version.

SERVES 2

- ¼ pound arugula leaves (about 6 cups)
- One 6-ounce can solid light tuna in olive oil, such as the Progresso brand, drained, with oil reserved (substitute tuna canned in soybean oil if you can't find the olive oil version)
- 1 cup grape tomato halves
- ½ small red onion, thinly sliced
- ¼ cup shredded ricotta salata or crumbled feta cheese
- Juice and zest of 1 lemon

In a large salad bowl, combine the arugula, tuna, grape tomatoes, red onion, and cheese.

To make the dressing, combine the lemon juice, zest, and reserved olive oil in a small bowl. Whisk to blend.

Drizzle the dressing over the salad and toss well to coat.

PER SERVING, ABOUT: Calories: 291, Protein: 30 g, Carbohydrate: 10 g, Dietary Fiber: 2 g, Total Fat: 15 g, Saturated Fat: 5 g, Cholesterol: 32 mg, Calcium: 204 mg, Sodium: 533 mg.

Curried Chicken, Apple, and Toasted Millet Salad

Millet, rich in magnesium, is considered a sacred grain by the Chinese. Here it adds texture and balances out this dish's nutrient mix.

SERVES 4

> ½ cup millet or bulgur wheat
>
> 1 cup fat-free chicken broth, such as Health Valley fat-free chicken broth or Pacific Foods low-sodium chicken broth, or water
>
> 1½ cups diced cooked skinless chicken breast
>
> 1 apple, cored and diced
>
> ½ cup thinly sliced celery
>
> ¼ cup currants
>
> 4 teaspoons reduced-sodium soy sauce
>
> 1 tablespoon rice vinegar
>
> ½ teaspoon curry powder
>
> Salt and freshly ground pepper

In a dry small saucepan set over a medium-low flame, toast the millet until it's golden, about 10 minutes, stirring frequently. (If using bulgur, do not toast.) Add the broth and bring the mixture to a boil.

Reduce the heat to low, cover the saucepan, and simmer the millet until it is tender, about 30 minutes (bulgur wheat takes 20 to 25 minutes). Transfer the cooked grain to a large bowl, fluff it with a fork, and let it cool.

Add the chicken, apple, celery, and currants to the cooled grain.

In a small bowl, mix the soy sauce, rice vinegar, and curry powder. Pour the dressing over the salad and mix thoroughly.

Season the salad with salt and pepper.

PER SERVING, ABOUT: Calories: 238, Protein: 20 g, Carbohydrate: 32 g, Dietary Fiber: 4 g, Total Fat: 3 g, Saturated Fat: 1 g, Cholesterol: 45 mg, Calcium: 27 mg, Sodium: 336 mg.

Chicken Salad with Pomegranate, Oranges, and Walnuts

This salad includes a double dose of pomegranate: both the juice and its seeds. Pomegranates are rich in antioxidants and have been shown to lower LDL ("bad") cholesterol.

SERVES 4

> 2½ cups mixed baby greens, baby arugula, or watercress
>
> 2 cups chopped cooked chicken breast
>
> 2 oranges, peeled and cut into segments
>
> ½ cup pomegranate seeds (if you can't find pomegranates, substitute ¼ cup dried cranberries)
>
> ½ cup toasted walnuts
>
> 1 tablespoon chopped chives
>
> ¼ cup pomegranate juice
>
> 2 tablespoons orange juice
>
> 2 tablespoons olive oil
>
> Salt and freshly ground pepper

In a large mixing bowl, combine the baby greens, chicken, oranges, pomegranate seeds, walnuts, and chives.

In a small bowl, whisk together the pomegranate juice, orange juice, and olive oil. Season with salt and pepper. Pour the dressing over the salad and toss the salad to combine.

PER SERVING, ABOUT: Calories: 346, Protein: 26 g, Carbohydrate: 21 g, Dietary Fiber: 3 g, Total Fat: 19 g, Saturated Fat: 3 g, Cholesterol: 60 mg, Calcium: 76 mg, Sodium: 64 mg.

Whole Wheat Pasta Salad
with Broccoli and Peanut Sauce

This dish is reminiscent of Chinese sesame noodles—only it's a lot leaner. It can also be served hot.

SERVES 4

> 5 tablespoons peanut butter
>
> 1 tablespoon rice vinegar
>
> 1 tablespoon water
>
> 1 tablespoon plus 1 teaspoon reduced-sodium soy sauce
>
> 1 teaspoon freshly squeezed lime juice
>
> 1 teaspoon minced garlic
>
> ⅛ teaspoon cayenne
>
> 4 cups broccoli florets and thinly sliced stems (about 1 pound)
>
> 8 ounces whole wheat fusilli, cooked

In a small bowl, combine the peanut butter, rice vinegar, water, soy sauce, lime juice, garlic, and cayenne. Set aside.

In a medium saucepan with a steamer insert, steam the broccoli over boiling water, covered, until the broccoli is tender yet crisp, 1 to 2 minutes.

Combine the broccoli and cooked pasta in a medium bowl, pour the peanut sauce over the mixture, and toss. Chill in the refrigerator and serve.

PER SERVING, ABOUT: Calories: 237, Protein: 12 g, Carbohydrate: 27 g, Dietary Fiber: 6 g, Total Fat: 10 g, Saturated Fat: 2 g, Cholesterol: 0 mg, Calcium: 64 mg, Sodium: 277 mg.

SANDWICHES AND WRAPS

Black Bean Chipotle Burger with Corn Salsa

Veggie burgers have come a long way. This variation on the theme has a smoky, spicy flavor and is topped with a confetti-like jumble of healthful vegetables.

SERVES 4

Corn Salsa

1 cup frozen corn kernels, such as Cascadian Farm organic, thawed

½ red bell pepper, seeded and diced

½ green bell pepper, seeded and diced

2 tablespoons diced red onion

2 tablespoons sliced fresh chives

Salt and freshly ground pepper

Tabasco sauce

Black Bean Chipotle Burger

Two 15-ounce cans black beans, drained and rinsed

2 tablespoons chopped cilantro

½ chipotle chile, rinsed and chopped

Salt and freshly ground pepper

Cornmeal for coating

3 tablespoons light mayonnaise

1–2 teaspoons adobo sauce from chipotle chiles

Nonstick cooking spray

4 whole wheat burger buns

Lettuce leaves and tomato slices

Blanch the corn in rapidly boiling salted water until the water returns to a boil. Drain and rinse the corn with cold water. Transfer it to a mixing bowl. Add the bell peppers, onion, and chives, and mix. Season the mixture with salt, pepper, and Tabasco.

Place half of the beans in a small bowl and mash them into a smooth paste. Stir in the remaining beans along with the cilantro and chipotle chile. Season this mixture with salt and pepper. Form it into 4 patties. Dip each patty in cornmeal to coat it lightly. Refrigerate the patties on a waxed paper–lined tray for at least 30 minutes.

Meanwhile, in a small bowl, blend the mayonnaise and adobo sauce. (It's very spicy, so taste-test before adding the entire 1–2 teaspoons.)

Coat a nonstick skillet with cooking spray. Heat the skillet over a medium flame. Carefully add the bean patties and sauté them for about 1 minute. Carefully turn the patties and sauté them for 1 minute longer, or until heated through.

Spread the bun bottoms with the mayonnaise mixture. Top them with lettuce, tomato, and the hot bean patties. Top each patty with corn salsa and cover it with the bun top.

Timesaver: Substitute Gardenburger Black Bean Chipotle Burgers or another bean- or soy-based veggie burger of your choice.

PER SERVING, ABOUT: Calories: 457, Protein: 23 g, Carbohydrate: 85 g, Dietary Fiber: 24 g, Total Fat: 5 g, Saturated Fat: 1 g, Cholesterol: 3 mg, Calcium: 148 mg, Sodium: 595 mg.

Chicken Tabbouleh Pitas

Tabbouleh is a great traditional Middle Eastern grain salad. In this recipe, chicken was added to bolster its protein content.

SERVES 4

> 2 cups fat-free chicken broth, such as Health Valley fat-free chicken broth or Pacific Foods low-sodium chicken broth
>
> 1 cup fine bulgur wheat
>
> Juice and zest of 1 lemon
>
> 2 tablespoons extra-virgin olive oil
>
> Salt and freshly ground pepper
>
> 1 cup chopped cooked chicken breast
>
> ½ cup packed finely chopped fresh parsley
>
> 2 green onions, finely chopped
>
> 1 cup Muir Glen Organic Fire Roasted Diced Tomatoes,* drained
>
> ⅔ cup diced cucumber
>
> 2 whole wheat pitas, halved

In a saucepan, bring the chicken broth to a boil. Slowly stir in the bulgur. Reduce the flame to low, cover the pan, and cook until the broth is absorbed, about 15 minutes. Transfer the bulgur to a large bowl to cool.

Meanwhile, in a small bowl, combine the lemon juice, lemon zest, olive oil, salt, and pepper. Add the chicken and toss well. Set the mixture aside.

In a large bowl, combine the parsley, green onion, tomatoes, and cucumber. Add the cooled bulgur and chicken with dressing. Toss the mixture well to combine. Serve in pita halves.

* If fire-roasted tomatoes are unavailable, use regular canned diced tomatoes.

PER SERVING, ABOUT: Calories: 271, Protein: 17 g, Carbohydrate: 32 g, Dietary Fiber: 5 g, Total Fat: 9 g, Saturated Fat: 1 g, Cholesterol: 30 mg, Calcium: 44 mg, Sodium: 480 mg.

Walnut Cannellini Wraps

This fiber-rich spread is the perfect base for a fast weekday lunch but can also be served as a stand-alone dip with cut-up vegetables or toasted pita chips.

SERVES 6

One 15-ounce can cannellini beans, drained and rinsed

½ cup walnuts

¼ cup packed fresh parsley leaves

3 tablespoons fresh lemon juice (juice of about 1 lemon)

2 tablespoons extra-virgin olive oil

1 clove garlic, minced

¼ teaspoon kosher salt

Freshly ground pepper

6 whole wheat flour tortillas, about 75 calories apiece

1 large carrot, peeled and shredded (about 1 cup)

1–2 packed cups arugula or baby spinach, washed well

Combine the beans, walnuts, parsley, lemon juice, olive oil, garlic, salt, and a few pinches of pepper in the bowl of a food processor; process the mixture until smooth and creamy. Season with additional salt and pepper. To make the wraps, spread the bean mixture evenly over each of the tortillas; layer the tortillas with the carrot and arugula. Roll the wrap, slice in half, and serve.

PER SERVING, ABOUT: Calories: 238, Protein: 9 g, Carbohydrate: 35 g, Dietary Fiber: 6 g, Total Fat: 11 g, Saturated Fat: 1 g, Cholesterol: 0 mg, Calcium: 71 mg, Sodium: 400 mg.

Whole Wheat Burritos with Black Beans, Brown Rice, Greens, and Corn Salsa

These burritos improve on the traditional recipe by substituting brown rice for white and adding Swiss chard, a good source of beta-carotene.

SERVES 4

- 1 bunch Swiss chard
- 2 tablespoons of water
- Four 10-inch fat-free whole wheat tortillas, about 75 calories apiece
- 2 cups warm cooked brown rice
- 2 cups black beans, drained, rinsed, and warmed
- Corn Salsa (see recipe on page 224)

Rinse the Swiss chard thoroughly and remove any tough stems. Coarsely chop the leaves. Place the leaves along with the water in a skillet over a medium flame and cover. Cook the leaves until they are wilted, about 2 minutes.

Heat the tortillas on a hot griddle or in a skillet set over a medium flame. Remove from heat.

Place ½ cup each of the brown rice and the beans in a strip down the center of each tortilla. Top each tortilla with some of the greens and the Corn Salsa. Fold the ends over the filling and roll up.

PER SERVING, ABOUT: Calories: 344, Protein: 15 g, Carbohydrate: 76 g, Dietary Fiber: 14 g, Total Fat: 2 g, Saturated Fat: 0 g, Cholesterol: 0 mg, Calcium: 82 mg, Sodium: 632 mg.

Southwestern Veggie Burgers Supreme

SERVES 4

Spice up store-bought veggie burgers with this easy and flavorful topping.

   ¼ cup light mayonnaise (no more than 50 calories and 5 g fat per tablespoon), such as Hellmann's Canola Cholesterol Free

   1 tablespoon chopped fresh cilantro

   1 tablespoon lime juice (the juice of ½ of a lime)

   ¼ teaspoon ground cumin

   ⅛ teaspoon chili powder

   Salt and freshly ground pepper

   4 whole wheat hamburger buns, lightly toasted

   4 soy-based vegetable burgers, cooked, such as Amy's Texas Burger, Boca All-American Flame Grilled, or Gardenburger Flame Grilled

   1 avocado, pitted and cut into thin slices

   4 slices tomato

   1 cup arugula

Combine the mayonnaise, cilantro, lime juice, cumin, and chili powder, and season with salt and pepper; mix until well blended. Spread the mixture evenly over the bottoms of the hamburger buns. Place each veggie burger on a bun half and top evenly with the avocado, tomato, and arugula. Cover each burger with the remaining bun half and serve.

PER SERVING, ABOUT: Calories: 367, Protein: 19 g, Carbohydrate: 37 g, Dietary Fiber: 11 g, Total Fat: 18 g, Saturated Fat: 2 g, Cholesterol: 5 mg, Calcium: 70 mg, Sodium: 603 mg.

ENTREES

Beef

Steak Tagliata with Peppers and Zucchini

You can whip up this impressive dish in under 25 minutes.

SERVES 4

> 3 tablespoons extra-virgin olive oil, such as Bertolli
>
> 1 clove garlic, minced
>
> 1 small yellow onion, finely diced
>
> 2 medium zucchini, finely diced
>
> 1 yellow and 1 red bell pepper, seeded and finely diced
>
> 2 tablespoons finely chopped lemon pulp
>
> 1 teaspoon grated lemon zest
>
> 3–4 tablespoons finely chopped fresh parsley
>
> ¼ teaspoon salt
>
> ⅛ teaspoon freshly ground black pepper
>
> 1 pound boneless sirloin or rib-eye steaks, 1 inch thick

In 12-inch nonstick skillet, heat the olive oil over medium heat. Sauté the garlic for 30 seconds, then add the onion to the pan. Sauté another 5 minutes, or until onion begins to soften. Add the zucchini and peppers and cook, stirring occasionally, until the vegetables are softened but still a little crisp, about 10 minutes.

To the skillet, add the lemon pulp, lemon zest, parsley, salt, and black pepper, and transfer to a bowl. Cover the bowl to keep the vegetables warm.

Season the steaks, if desired, with salt and pepper. In the same skillet, cook the steaks for 4 to 8 minutes, or until desired doneness, turning once. Let the steaks stand for 5 minutes, then slice and serve with the vegetables.

PER SERVING, ABOUT: Calories: 360, Protein: 27 g, Carbohydrate: 11 g, Dietary Fiber: 3 g, Total Fat: 24 g, Saturated Fat: 7 g, Cholesterol: 100 mg, Calcium: 52 mg, Sodium: 210 mg.

Flank Steak with Chimichurri Topping

Chimichurri is an herb sauce served with practically everything in Argentina. Although it's oil-based, it's extremely flavorful—a little dab will do you.

SERVES 4

> 1 cup parsley leaves, about 1 bunch, stemmed
>
> 4 cloves garlic, roughly chopped
>
> 2 shallots, roughly chopped
>
> 1 small jalapeño, stemmed, seeded, and roughly chopped (optional)
>
> 3 tablespoons extra-virgin olive oil
>
> 2 tablespoons freshly squeezed lime juice
>
> ½ teaspoon crushed red pepper flakes
>
> ¼ teaspoon ground cumin
>
> ¼ teaspoon salt
>
> 1 pound flank steak

In a food processor, combine the parsley, garlic, shallots, jalapeño (if using), olive oil, lime juice, pepper flakes, cumin, and salt. Process the mixture with on-off bursts until the contents are coarsely chopped. Scrape down the sides of the bowl with a rubber spatula. Process the mixture a few seconds more until finely chopped.

Transfer the mixture to a small bowl, cover it, and let stand for at least 30 minutes.

Grill the steak over hot coals or broil it until done as desired. Slice the steak on the diagonal and serve it drizzled with the topping.

PER SERVING, ABOUT: Calories: 265, Protein: 24 g, Carbohydrate: 4 g, Dietary Fiber: 1 g, Total Fat: 17 g, Saturated Fat: 4 g, Cholesterol: 64 mg, Calcium: 38 mg, Sodium: 393 mg.

Spicy Beef Fajitas with Fire-Roasted Salsa Guacamole

This guacamole is so good, it'll replace any of your old recipes. It's made with
lots of chopped veggies, which enhances its flavor and makes it less caloric.

SERVES 6

Marinade

3 tablespoons canola oil

3 tablespoons freshly squeezed lime juice

2 tablespoons Worcestershire sauce

1 teaspoon pepper

½ teaspoon minced garlic

Filling

1¼-pound flank steak, cut into 3 x ¼-inch strips*

2 tablespoons canola oil

1 large green pepper, cut into julienne strips (1 cup)

1 large red pepper, cut into julienne strips (1 cup)

1 medium onion, thinly sliced (½ cup)

18 small corn tortillas, about 42 calories each

6 servings Fire-Roasted Salsa Guacamole (see the following recipe)

In medium nonreactive bowl, combine all of the marinade ingredients; mix
them well. Add the steak, turning to coat all of its sides. Cover; refrigerate for at
least 3 hours, turning the steak occasionally. Drain off marinade and discard.

In a 12-inch skillet, heat the oil over high heat for 1 minute. Add the
marinated steak, green pepper, red pepper, and onion; stir-fry the contents
for 5 minutes, or until the steak is no longer pink and the vegetables are
crisp-tender. Drain.

Heat the tortillas as directed on the package. Serve tortillas alongside steak
and pepper mix and Fire-Roasted Salsa Guacamole.

PER SERVING, ABOUT: Calories: 433, Protein: 28 g, Carbohydrate: 44 g, Dietary
Fiber: 8 g, Total Fat: 18 g, Saturated Fat: 4 g, Cholesterol: 35 mg, Calcium:
175 mg, Sodium: 180 mg.

* For easier slicing, place the steak in a freezer for 1 hour, or until firm but not
frozen; slice the steak thinly across the grain of the meat.

Fire-Roasted Salsa Guacamole

You can also serve this with baked tortilla chips or fresh vegetables.

SERVES 12 (¼ CUP EACH)

Salsa

One 14½-ounce can Muir Glen Organic Fire Roasted or plain diced
  tomatoes, well drained

¼ cup chopped onion

2 tablespoons chopped fresh cilantro

¼ teaspoon coarse salt (kosher or sea salt)

1 clove garlic, finely chopped

1 small jalapeño, stemmed, seeded, and finely chopped

Guacamole

3 large ripe avocados (about 1½ pounds), pitted and peeled

2 tablespoons freshly squeezed lime juice

½ teaspoon coarse salt (kosher or sea salt)

½ teaspoon red pepper sauce

1 clove garlic, finely chopped

In a medium bowl, stir the salsa ingredients together.

In another medium bowl, coarsely mash the avacados. Stir in the remaining
guacamole ingredients. Spoon the guacamole into a shallow serving bowl;
top with salsa.

PER SERVING, ABOUT: Calories: 92, Protein: 1 g, Carbohydrate: 7 g, Dietary
Fiber: 4 g, Total Fat: 7 g, Saturated Fat: 1 g, Cholesterol: 0 mg, Calcium: 14 mg,
Sodium: 201 mg.

Chicken

Chicken with Artichokes and Melted Lemons

Simple yet elegant, this is the kind of dish that's perfect for entertaining.

SERVES 4

> 2 teaspoons olive oil
>
> 4 pieces boneless, skinless chicken breasts (about 1 pound)
>
> Juice of 1 lemon
>
> ¾ cup chicken stock or canned low-sodium chicken broth, such as Health Valley no-salt-added chicken broth or Pacific Foods low-sodium chicken broth
>
> 1 lemon, thinly sliced
>
> 2 tablespoons capers with juice
>
> One 14-ounce can quartered artichoke hearts, drained
>
> Salt and freshly ground black pepper

Heat the olive oil in an 8-inch skillet over medium-high heat. When the olive oil is heated, swirl it to cover the bottom of pan. Add the chicken breasts and sear them until browned. Turn the chicken breasts and brown them on the other side. Remove the chicken to a plate and increase the heat to high. Deglaze the pan with the lemon juice, scraping up any browned bits into the sauce.

Add the stock and bring to a simmer. Add the lemon slices to the pan, reduce the heat to medium, and place the chicken breasts on top of the lemon slices. Add the capers, cover, reduce the heat to medium, and cook, covered, for 10 minutes. Remove the lid and add the drained artichoke hearts. Cover and continue cooking for 5 minutes, or until the breasts are cooked through.

Remove the chicken to a warm plate. Increase the temperature and reduce the sauce to a glaze. Taste the sauce and adjust the seasoning with salt and pepper as needed. Just a little salt will reduce the acidity of the lemons, capers, and artichokes and balance the flavors. Serve the chicken with the artichoke hearts, capers, and melted lemons drizzled with the glaze.

PER SERVING, ABOUT: Calories: 186, Protein: 29 g, Carbohydrate: 34 g, Dietary Fiber: 6 g, Total Fat: 4 g, Saturated Fat: 1 g, Cholesterol: 66 mg, Calcium: 79 mg, Sodium: 552 mg.

Chicken Sausage Jambalaya

This southern classic gets a healthy update with brown rice and chicken (instead of pork) sausage. Serve with hot pepper sauce, if desired.

SERVES 4

 1 tablespoon olive oil

 1½ cups sliced smoked chicken sausage or chicken andouille

 1 red bell pepper, seeded and chopped

 1 large onion, chopped

 1 cup chopped celery

 2 cloves garlic, minced

 ½ cup chopped parsley

 1 teaspoon dried basil

 1 teaspoon oregano

 1 bay leaf

 2 cups no-salt-added diced tomatoes, canned (such as Muir Glen organic no-salt-added diced tomatoes) or in a carton

 1 cup fat-free chicken broth, such as Health Valley fat-free chicken broth or Pacific Foods low-sodium chicken broth

 3 cups cooked brown rice

 Salt and freshly ground black pepper

 ½ cup thinly sliced green onions

In a pot set over a medium-high flame, heat the olive oil. Add the sausages and cook them until they begin to brown, stirring occasionally, about 7 minutes.

Add the bell pepper, onion, and celery. Sauté, stirring often, until the onion is golden, about 10 minutes. Add the garlic, parsley, basil, oregano, and bay leaf. Cook, stirring several times, 2 minutes longer.

Add the tomatoes, breaking up into pieces with a spoon. Add the chicken broth and bring to a boil. Cover, reduce the heat, and simmer for 10 minutes. Stir in the rice, cover, and simmer for 10 minutes longer. Season with salt and black pepper. Remove the bay leaf. Serve sprinkled with green onions.

PER SERVING, ABOUT: Calories: 355, Protein: 13 g, Carbohydrate: 48 g, Dietary Fiber: 8 g, Total Fat: 13 g, Saturated Fat: 3 g, Cholesterol: 51 mg, Calcium: 119 mg, Sodium: 518 mg.

Whole Roasted Chicken with Citrus and Whole Grain Bread Crumbs

A flavorful bread-crumb crust elevates this easy chicken dish from ordinary to extraordinary.

SERVES 4

1 whole chicken, about 3½–4 pounds

¾ teaspoon salt

Freshly ground pepper

1 orange, zested and cut into 8 wedges, zest reserved

1 whole lemon, zested and cut into 8 wedges, zest reserved

¼ cup whole grain bread crumbs

3 tablespoons grated Parmesan cheese

6–8 large cloves garlic, minced

2 teaspoons chopped fresh thyme

2 tablespoons olive oil

Preheat the oven to 425 degrees F. and position a rack in the lower third of oven.

Rinse the chicken in warm water, then dry it, inside and out, with paper towels. Trim any extra fat away from around the cavity, especially from around the tail end.

Sprinkle ½ teaspoon of salt and some pepper on the outside and cavity, and place 4 of the orange and 4 of the lemon wedges inside, squeezing them a little as you put them in.

Fold the wing tips under the body of the chicken. Tie the ends of the drumsticks together with kitchen twine. Place the chicken breast up on a roasting rack in a roasting pan. Roast for 15 minutes, then lower the heat to 375 degrees F. and roast for 15 minutes longer.

Meanwhile, in a small bowl, create a paste by combining the orange and lemon zests, bread crumbs, Parmesan, garlic, thyme, and olive oil. Season with remaining ¼ teaspoon of salt and some pepper. Set aside.

Remove the chicken from the oven; let it stand a few minutes to cool slightly. Carefully run a knife under the skin, and pull the skin away from the breast and legs with your fingers. Discard the skin. Squeeze the juice from the remaining orange and lemon pieces over the chicken. Apply the paste by rubbing it into the outside of the chicken. Return the chicken to the oven and roast it for another 45 minutes, basting several times with pan drippings, taking care not to dislodge the crumb paste.

To test for doneness, carefully slice into the joint at the thigh and check if the juices run clear. If not, return to the oven. When done, remove the chicken from the oven, and let it rest on a cooling rack for at least 10 minutes before carving. Discard the wings.

PER SERVING, ABOUT: Calories: 375, Protein: 41 g, Carbohydrate: 11 g, Dietary Fiber: 2 g, Total Fat: 18 g, Saturated Fat: 4 g, Cholesterol: 116 mg, Calcium: 101 mg, Sodium: 663 mg.

Pork

Spicy Pork Tenderloin with Citrus Salsa

Tenderloin is one of the leanest cuts of pork. Here it's rubbed with a spicy paste and topped with a tangy salsa. Serve it with something simple on the side, such as rice pilaf and grilled asparagus.

SERVES 4

      1 tablespoon cumin seeds

      1 tablespoon chili powder

      1 teaspoon dried oregano

      1 teaspoon coriander seeds

      ¼ teaspoon coarse salt (kosher or sea salt)

      1 pound pork tenderloin

      1 large or 2 small oranges, peeled and diced* (about 1 cup)

      1 grapefruit, peeled and diced* (about ¾ cup)

      ½ cup chopped dried cranberries

      ½ cup chopped cilantro

      ¼ cup minced red onion

      1 small jalapeño, stemmed, seeded, and minced (optional)

In a dry skillet set over medium heat, toast the cumin, chili powder, oregano, coriander, and salt, stirring constantly, until aroma is released, about 30 seconds. Cool slightly, then transfer the mixture to a blender (the container must be completely dry) or coffee grinder and process for about 15 seconds.

Put the spice mixture evenly all over tenderloin. Wrap the mixture in plastic wrap and refrigerate it for several hours or up to overnight.

To make the salsa, combine the orange, grapefruit, cranberries, cilantro, red onion, and jalapeño in a medium bowl. Toss the mixture to combine. Cover and refrigerate it until 30 minutes before serving time.

Grill the tenderloin over medium-hot coals, turning several times, until the internal temperature registers 145 degrees F., about 20 minutes.

Alternatively, the tenderloin can be roasted in a preheated 400-degree oven until the internal temperature registers 145 degrees F., about 20 minutes.

Let the tenderloin rest, covered with foil, about 5 minutes. Cut the tenderloin into thick slices and serve it with the salsa.

* To peel the orange and grapefruit, set each fruit on its side on a cutting board and slice off about ½ inch from both ends. Turn the fruit so it rests on a cut side, and following the curve of the fruit, cut from top to bottom, turning the fruit and cutting away both the peel and pith all the way around. Turn the fruit over and cut in same manner to remove any remaining peel or pith. Holding the fruit over a bowl to catch the juices, cut between the pith lines to remove individual segments; then chop.

PER SERVING, ABOUT: Calories: 255, Protein: 26 g, Carbohydrate: 28 g, Dietary Fiber: 5 g, Total Fat: 5 g, Saturated Fat: 1 g, Cholesterol: 74 mg, Calcium: 77 mg, Sodium: 202 mg.

Pork Chop and Cabbage Bake

You can make this hearty dish any time of year, but it's particularly nice when the weather is cold.

SERVES 4

1 tablespoon fennel seeds

1 tablespoon fresh rosemary leaves or 1 teaspoon dried rosemary

3 cloves garlic, roughly chopped

½ teaspoon coarsely ground pepper

½ teaspoon coarse salt (kosher or sea salt)

4 boneless pork loin chops (1 pound)

1 cup thinly sliced onion

1½ cups reduced-sodium chicken broth, such as Health Valley no-salt-added chicken broth or Pacific Foods low-sodium chicken broth

Half of a 16-ounce package of coleslaw mix (about 5 cups)

1 Granny Smith apple, cored and cut into 16 wedges

Place the fennel, rosemary, garlic, pepper, and salt in a blender and process 30 seconds, stopping twice to scrape up the mixture. Pat the fennel mixture on one side of each chop. Cover the chops and let stand for 30 minutes.

Preheat the oven to 375 degrees F.

In a 10-inch iron skillet or other ovenproof skillet set over high heat, combine the onion and ½ cup of the chicken broth. Bring the mixture to a boil. Cook and stir until the broth is evaporated and the onion loses its shine, about 8 minutes. Add the remaining broth. Bring the mixture to a boil. Add the coleslaw mix and apples and stir to combine.

Remove the pan from the heat and arrange the pork chops in a single layer over the cabbage. Place in the oven and bake until the meat registers 145 degrees F. on a meat thermometer, about 15 minutes. Remove the chops from the oven and cover them loosely with foil. Let stand for 10 minutes before serving.

PER SERVING, ABOUT: Calories: 237, Protein: 27 g, Carbohydrate: 15 g, Dietary Fiber: 4 g, Total Fat: 8 g, Saturated Fat: 3 g, Cholesterol: 62 mg, Calcium: 79 mg, Sodium: 398 mg.

Seafood

Grilled Tuna with Zesty Green Sauce

The green in this fat-free Asian sauce comes from jalapeño pepper. To lower the sauce's heat, remove the pepper's ribs and seeds before mincing. Since different varieties of tuna are safer than others, check www.oceansalive.org for an update before you buy.

SERVES 4

> 2 tablespoons reduced-sodium soy sauce
>
> 1 tablespoon peeled, minced fresh ginger
>
> 2 tablespoons freshly squeezed lime juice
>
> 2 tablespoons orange juice
>
> ¼ cup chopped fresh cilantro
>
> 2 teaspoons honey
>
> ½ teaspoon minced jalapeño, or to taste
>
> 1 clove garlic, finely minced
>
> Four 4-ounce tuna steaks or any thick-cut fish steaks, such as Pacific halibut or swordfish
>
> 1 teaspoon sesame oil
>
> Salt and freshly ground pepper

In a small saucepan, combine the soy sauce, ginger, lime and orange juices, cilantro, honey, jalapeño, and garlic. Set aside.

Prepare a barbecue by heating coals to medium-high heat, or preheat the broiler. Brush the tuna with the oil and sprinkle with salt and pepper. Grill or broil the fish until just opaque in the center, about 4 minutes per side. Set aside, tented with foil.

Meanwhile, warm the sauce over a low flame until it is just simmering. Do not allow the sauce to boil.

Spoon the sauce over the grilled fish.

PER SERVING, ABOUT: Calories: 159, Protein: 28 g, Carbohydrate: 6 g, Dietary Fiber: 0 g, Total Fat: 2 g, Saturated Fat: 0 g, Cholesterol: 51 mg, Calcium: 24 mg, Sodium: 324 mg.

Grilled Snapper with Eggplant, Squash, and Potatoes

This dish has a slightly different twist: lemon halves are grilled before
they're squeezed over the fish.

SERVES 4

2 cups of water

½ teaspoon salt

1 cup peeled, diced boiling potatoes (about 2 potatoes)

2 teaspoons olive oil

2 teaspoons minced garlic

1 cup eggplant, diced (about ½ small eggplant)

1 cup zucchini, diced (about 1 small zucchini)

1 cup yellow squash, diced (about 1 small squash)

3 cups fresh diced plum tomatoes (about 4 tomatoes)

3 tablespoons fresh or 1 tablespoon dried oregano, minced

Nonstick cooking spray

2 lemons, cut into halves

1 pound fresh snapper or another firm-fleshed white fish, such as tilapia

Salt and freshly ground pepper

Preheat the grill to a medium setting.

Heat a large, straight-sided skillet. Add 2 cups of water and ½ teaspoon salt.
Bring the water to a boil. Add the diced potatoes and blanch them in the
boiling water for 3 minutes, just until they start to soften. Drain the
potatoes, reserving the cooking liquid. Set the potatoes aside.

To the same pan, add the olive oil and heat it through over medium heat.
Swirl the oil to cover the bottom of the pan. Sauté the garlic until it's
fragrant, about 1 minute. Add the eggplant, zucchini, and squash, and sauté
the vegetables for another 5 minutes. Add the diced tomatoes and oregano
and cook another 5 minutes, until the vegetables are heated through and
starting to fall apart. If the pan is dry, add a little of the reserved potato
cooking liquid.

While the vegetables are cooking, grill the lemons and fish. Spray the grill with nonstick spray. Place the lemon halves, cut side down, on the hottest part of the grill, and cook them until they are charred and fragrant. Season the fish on both sides with salt and pepper. Grill the fish, skin side down, with the grill covered, about 6 minutes or just until the fish is starting to flake.

To serve, place a bed of the vegetables on the plate, top this with a piece of the fish, and squeeze the charred lemon over all.

PER SERVING, ABOUT: Calories: 215, Protein: 27 g, Carbohydrate: 21 g, Dietary Fiber: 7 g, Total Fat: 5 g, Saturated Fat: 1 g, Cholesterol: 42 mg, Calcium: 135 mg, Sodium: 93 mg.

Lemon and Herb Grilled Trout

Evocative of a seaside taverna in Greece, this dish is quick, easy, and delicious enough for company.

SERVES 4

> 4 whole trout, cleaned, with head and tail left on
>
> ¼ cup extra-virgin olive oil, such as Bertolli
>
> 4 teaspoons finely chopped fresh thyme or oregano leaves
>
> 4 teaspoons chopped fresh parsley
>
> ½ teaspoon kosher salt
>
> 8 thin slices lemon

Rinse the trout inside and out; pat dry. Generously brush each trout, inside and out, with the olive oil. Sprinkle the inside of each trout with 1 teaspoon thyme, 1 teaspoon parsley, and salt; put 2 slices of lemon in each trout. If desired, use several toothpicks to seal fish closed. Grill or broil trout, turning once, for 14 minutes, or until fish flakes with a fork. To serve, arrange the trout on serving platter.

PER SERVING, ABOUT: Calories: 344, Protein: 43 g, Carbohydrate: 0 g, Dietary Fiber: 0 g, Total Fat: 18 g, Saturated Fat: 4 g, Cholesterol: 120 mg, Calcium: 144 mg, Sodium: 313 mg.

Tuscan Cod and Mussels in Light Vegetable Broth

A beautiful dish; the white cod is set off by the bright red and green sauce.

SERVES 4

3 tablespoons extra-virgin olive oil, such as Bertolli

1 large sweet onion, such as Walla Walla or Vidalia, coarsely chopped

1 medium zucchini, coarsely chopped

½ teaspoon salt

1 clove garlic, chopped

One 14½-ounce can whole peeled plum tomatoes, undrained and chopped, no-salt-added or low-sodium (about 20 mg sodium per ½ cup)

¼ cup dry white wine, fish broth, or vegetable broth

1 pound cod fillet, cut into 4-inch pieces

1 dozen mussels, well scrubbed

2 tablespoons finely chopped fresh parsley (optional)

In a deep 12-inch nonstick skillet, heat the olive oil over medium-high heat and cook the onion, zucchini, and salt, stirring occasionally, for about 10 minutes. Add the garlic and cook for 30 seconds. Stir in the tomatoes and wine or broth and simmer for 2 minutes.

Arrange the cod in the skillet. Simmer the fish, covered, for 6 minutes and add mussels. Cook for another 4 minutes, or until the fish flakes with a fork and the mussel shells open. Discard any unopened shells. Sprinkle with parsley. Season to taste with additional salt if desired.

PER SERVING, ABOUT: Calories: 27 g, Protein: 28 g, Carbohydrate: 12 g, Dietary Fiber: 3 g, Total Fat: 12 g, Saturated Fat: 2 g, Cholesterol: 55 mg, Calcium: 57 mg, Sodium: 532 mg.

Fire-Roasted Tomato-Shrimp Veracruz

The 15 minutes it takes to prepare this dish belie its complex flavors. The surprising taste comes from a mix of jalapeño, thyme, and orange peel. Serve over brown rice or whole wheat couscous.

SERVES 4

> 1 tablespoon olive oil
>
> 1 pound medium raw shrimp, shelled and deveined, tails removed (if desired)
>
> 4 medium green onions, sliced (about ¼ cup)
>
> 1 medium fresh jalapeño or serrano chile, stemmed, seeded, and finely chopped
>
> 1 teaspoon grated orange zest
>
> 1 teaspoon chopped fresh thyme leaves or ½ teaspoon dried thyme leaves
>
> One 14½-ounce can Muir Glen Organic Fire Roasted Diced Tomatoes, undrained*

In a 12-inch skillet, heat the olive oil over medium-high heat. Cook the shrimp, green onions, chile, orange zest, and thyme in the oil for 1 minute, stirring frequently.

Stir in the tomatoes. Heat the mixture until it boils. Reduce the heat; simmer, uncovered, for about 5 minutes, or until shrimp are pink and firm and sauce is slightly thickened, stirring occasionally.

*If fire-roasted tomatoes are unavailable, use regular canned diced tomatoes.

PER SERVING, ABOUT: Calories: 180, Protein: 24 g, Carbohydrate: 7 g, Dietary Fiber: 1 g, Total Fat: 5 g, Saturated Fat: 1 g, Cholesterol: 172 mg, Calcium: 88 mg, Sodium: 400 mg.

Roasted Scallops with Tomato Salsa

Tender hot scallops pair gorgeously with cool bright red salsa.

SERVES 4

2 large tomatoes, seeded and chopped

6 kalamata or oil-cured olives, pitted and sliced

4 tablespoons extra-virgin olive oil, such as Bertolli

1 tablespoon finely chopped basil or oregano leaves or ½ teaspoon of
   dried basil or oregano leaves, crushed

2 teaspoons balsamic vinegar

1 clove garlic, finely chopped

½ teaspoon salt

¼ teaspoon ground black pepper

1 pound sea scallops

Preheat oven to 450 degrees F.

In a medium bowl, combine the tomatoes, olives, 2 tablespoons of olive oil,
basil, vinegar, garlic, ¼ teaspoon of salt, and ⅛ teaspoon of pepper. Let the
mixture stand for 10 minutes.

Meanwhile, in another medium bowl, toss the scallops with the remaining
2 tablespoons of olive oil, ¼ teaspoon of salt, and ⅛ teaspoon of pepper. In
a shallow roasting pan or jelly roll pan, arrange the scallops. Roast them for
10 minutes or until the scallops turn opaque. Serve the tomato salsa with
the hot scallops.

PER SERVING, ABOUT: Calories: 246, Protein: 20 g, Carbohydrate: 7 g, Dietary
Fiber: 1 g, Total Fat: 15 g, Saturated Fat: 2 g, Cholesterol: 37 mg, Calcium:
43 mg, Sodium: 477 mg.

Pasta, Stews, Risotto, and Pizza

Whole Wheat Penne with Fresh Pea Pesto

Peas give this pesto a lively flavor and allow you to cut down on oil (and forgo the cheese) usually included in pesto recipes.

SERVES 4

   1 cup freshly shelled peas (about 14 ounces) or 1 cup of thawed frozen shelled peas, such as Cascadian Farm organic

   ¾ cup fat-free chicken or vegetable broth, such as Health Valley fat-free chicken broth, Pacific Foods low-sodium chicken broth, or Health Valley fat-free vegetable broth

   2 tablespoons toasted pine nuts

   1 cup loosely packed basil leaves

   ½ cup loosely packed mint leaves

   2 garlic cloves, chopped

   2 tablespoons of extra-virgin olive oil

   Salt and freshly ground pepper

   12 ounces whole wheat penne rigate, cooked

In a small saucepan, combine the peas and broth. Bring to a boil, then reduce the heat, cover, and simmer the peas for 5 minutes, or until they're tender. If using frozen peas, cook according to package directions. Cool slightly.

In a blender, combine the peas and broth with the pine nuts, basil, mint, and garlic. Process to blend. With the blender running, slowly drizzle in the olive oil. Season with salt and pepper. Pour the pesto over the hot cooked pasta and toss to coat.

PER SERVING, ABOUT: Calories: 430, Protein: 14 g, Carbohydrate: 67 g, Dietary Fiber: 10 g, Total Fat: 13 g, Saturated Fat: 1 g, Cholesterol: 0 mg, Calcium: 67 mg, Sodium: 22 mg.

Broccoli Mac 'n' Cheese

The ultimate comfort food gets a healthy makeover with broccoli and whole wheat pasta.

SERVES 6 (1⅓ CUPS EACH)

> 8 ounces uncooked whole wheat penne pasta (2⅓ cups)
>
> 1 small red bell pepper, coarsely chopped (about 1 cup)
>
> One 24-ounce bag Green Giant frozen broccoli and three-cheese sauce
>
> 2 cups cubed cooked skinless chicken breast
>
> ¼ cup nonfat milk
>
> ⅛ teaspoon cayenne pepper
>
> ⅓ cup plain dry bread crumbs
>
> 3 tablespoons shredded Parmesan cheese
>
> ½ teaspoon Italian seasoning
>
> 1 tablespoon olive oil

Preheat the oven to 375 degrees F.

Grease a 13 x 9-inch baking dish. Cook the pasta as directed on the package, adding the bell pepper during the last 3 minutes of cooking time. Drain the pasta and return it to the saucepan.

Meanwhile, cook the broccoli and cheese sauce as directed on the package. Stir the cooked broccoli mixture, chicken, milk, and cayenne pepper into the pasta. Pour the pasta mixture into the baking dish.

In a small bowl, stir together the bread crumbs, Parmesan cheese, and Italian seasoning; stir in the olive oil, using a fork. Sprinkle the bread-crumb mixture over the top of the pasta mixture.

Bake for 15 to 20 minutes, or until the top is golden brown and the pasta is hot.

PER SERVING, ABOUT: Calories: 302, Protein: 22 g, Carbohydrate: 36 g, Dietary Fiber: 6 g, Total Fat: 8 g, Saturated Fat: 2 g, Cholesterol: 37 mg, Calcium: 106 mg, Sodium: 508 mg.

Pepper and Olive Tomato Sauce

Use this sauce on whole wheat pasta, or to top chicken, fish, beef, or pork.

SERVES 8 (¼ CUP EACH)

> 1 tablespoon olive oil
>
> 1 medium sweet onion, chopped (½ cup)
>
> 2 cloves garlic, finely chopped
>
> ½ medium red bell pepper, coarsely chopped (½ cup)
>
> ½ medium yellow bell pepper, coarsely chopped (½ cup)
>
> One 28-ounce can whole peeled tomatoes, such as Muir Glen organic, undrained and cut up
>
> 2 tablespoons tomato paste, such as Muir Glen organic
>
> ¼ teaspoon crushed red pepper
>
> ½ cup pitted and sliced kalamata olives

In a 10-inch skillet, heat the olive oil over medium heat. Cook the onion, garlic, and bell peppers in the oil for 4 to 5 minutes, stirring frequently, until crisp-tender. Stir in the tomatoes, tomato paste, and crushed red pepper. Heat the mixture until it boils.

Reduce the heat; simmer for 20 to 25 minutes or until thickened, stirring occasionally. Stir in the olives.

PER SERVING, ABOUT: Calories: 66, Protein: 1 g, Carbohydrate: 8 g, Dietary Fiber: 1 g, Total Fat: 3 g, Saturated Fat: 0 g, Cholesterol: 0 mg, Calcium: 23 mg, Sodium: 305 mg.

Mushroom Barley Risotto

Risotto made with barley is richer in fiber than versions made with Arborio rice. This dish also tastes great with asparagus instead or mushrooms.

SERVES 4

4 cups fat-free chicken or vegetable broth, such as Health Valley fat-free
  chicken broth, Pacific Foods low-sodium chicken broth, or Health
  Valley fat-free vegetable broth

2 tablespoons olive oil

1 small onion, chopped

¾ cup pearl barley, sorted and rinsed

⅓ cup dry white wine

½ pound portobello mushrooms, trimmed and sliced

2 tablespoons chopped shallots

2 tablespoons chopped fresh basil

Salt and freshly ground pepper

3 tablespoons grated Parmesan cheese

In a saucepan, bring the broth to a boil. Cover the pan and turn off the
heat.

Heat 1 tablespoon of the olive oil in a deep skillet over a medium flame.
Add the onion and sauté until soft. Reduce the heat to low. Add the barley
and stir it to coat with oil. Add the wine and cook, stirring, until wine is
absorbed. Add the hot broth, ½ cup at a time, stirring frequently and
adding ½ cup more of broth each time the previous addition is almost
absorbed. This should take about 30 minutes (you may have a little broth
left over). If the barley is not yet tender and all the broth is gone, add a little
water and cook until tender.

Put the remaining 1 tablespoon of the olive oil in a skillet over a medium-
high flame. Add the mushrooms and shallots and sauté until the
mushrooms are golden and the shallots are soft, about 5 minutes. (If the
mixture begins to stick, remove the skillet from the flame and spray the
mushrooms with nonstick cooking spray. Return the skillet to the heat
and cook until the mushrooms are golden and the shallots are soft.)

Stir the mushroom mixture and basil into the barley. Season with salt and
pepper. Serve immediately, sprinkled with Parmesan cheese.

PER SERVING, ABOUT: Calories: 257, Protein: 8 g, Carbohydrate: 36 g, Dietary
Fiber: 7 g, Total Fat: 8 g, Saturated Fat: 2 g, Cholesterol: 3 mg, Calcium: 66 mg,
Sodium: 167 mg.

Shrimp and Edamame Rotini

Edamame up the protein content of this dish while adding color and a slightly nutty flavor.

SERVES 5

> 8 ounces (about 3 cups) of dry whole wheat rotini or whole wheat blend rotini, such as fiber-enriched Barilla PLUS or Barilla Whole Grain
>
> 1½ cups frozen shelled edamame, thawed
>
> 1 tablespoon olive oil
>
> 4 cloves garlic, minced
>
> 1 pound large raw shrimp, shelled and deveined
>
> One 15-ounce can diced tomatoes
>
> ⅓ cup grated Parmesan cheese
>
> 3 tablespoons chopped fresh parsley
>
> Salt and pepper to taste

Cook the rotini in a large saucepan according to the package directions. Add the edamame for the last 5 minutes of cooking. When the pasta and edamame are done, drain and return to the saucepan.

While the pasta is cooking, heat the olive oil in a large nonstick skillet over medium heat. Add the garlic and cook until golden, 30 seconds to 1 minute. Add the shrimp and cook over high heat for 1 minute per side; add the diced tomatoes and bring to a boil. Lower the heat and simmer for an additional 2 minutes.

Combine the shrimp mixture with the cooked pasta and edamame. Toss with the Parmesan cheese and parsley. Season with salt and pepper.

PER SERVING, ABOUT: Calories: 486, Protein: 43 g, Carbohydrate: 58 g, Dietary Fiber: 10 g, Total Fat: 12 g, Saturated Fat: 3 g, Cholesterol: 180 mg, Calcium: 214 mg, Sodium: 537 mg.

Baked Pasta with Pumpkin and Spinach

Think baked ziti with major health twists: five times your daily vitamin A requirement in the form of healthy carotenes, 160 percent of your requirement of bone-strengthening vitamin K. And Barilla Whole Grain offers up five times the fiber of regular pasta.

SERVES 4

> 8 ounces Barilla Whole Grain Rotini
>
> 1⅓ cups fat-free ricotta
>
> 4 cups raw spinach
>
> ½ cup minced onion
>
> 2 cloves minced garlic
>
> 2 cups Libby's canned pumpkin
>
> ⅛ teaspoon ground nutmeg
>
> ¼ teaspoon salt
>
> Pepper to taste
>
> ¼ cup grated Parmesan cheese

Preheat oven to 375 degrees F.

Cook the rotini in a large saucepan according to the package directions. Drain thoroughly.

While pasta is cooking, combine ricotta, spinach, onion, garlic, pumpkin, nutmeg, salt, and pepper. Add drained pasta to ricotta mixture.

Spray a 9- or 10-inch baking pan with oil and place pasta mixture in pan. Top with Parmesan. Bake for 20 minutes. Turn oven up to broil and broil for 1 to 3 minutes, until top is bubbly and brown. Serve immediately.

PER SERVING, ABOUT: Calories: 382, Protein: 26 g, Carbohydrate: 60 g, Dietary Fiber: 13 g, Total Fat: 6 g, Saturated Fat: 2 g, Cholesterol: 18 mg, Calcium: 467 mg, Sodium: 474 mg.

Vegetarian Chili

Pair this with a cup of brown rice and you've got a highly nutritious, very satisfying 550-calorie dinner.

SERVES 4

1 tablespoon canola oil

1 large onion, chopped (1 cup)

1 medium green bell pepper, chopped (1 cup)

4 cloves garlic, finely chopped

2 fresh jalapeño or serrano chiles, seeded, finely chopped

Two 15-ounce cans black beans, preferably no-salt-added or reduced-
sodium, drained and rinsed

Two 14½-ounce cans Muir Glen organic Fire Roasted or plain diced
tomatoes, undrained

1½ cups water

1 tablespoon chili powder

1 teaspoon ground cumin

½ teaspoon coarse salt (kosher or sea salt)

1 cup frozen sweet corn, such as Cascadian Farm organic

Sour cream or plain yogurt, if desired

Shredded cheddar cheese, if desired

Chopped fresh cilantro, if desired

In a 4-quart saucepan, heat the oil over medium heat. Cook the onion, bell
pepper, garlic, and chiles in the oil 5 to 7 minutes, stirring frequently, until
tender.

Stir in the black beans, tomatoes, water, chili powder, cumin, and salt.
Heat the mixture until it boils. Reduce the heat; cover and simmer for
30 minutes, stirring occasionally. Stir in the corn. Heat until it boils. Reduce
the heat; simmer, uncovered, for 5 minutes longer.

Top each serving with sour cream, cheese, and cilantro.

PER SERVING, ABOUT: Calories: 330, Protein: 17 g, Carbohydrate: 59 g, Dietary
Fiber: 15 g, Total Fat: 4 g, Saturated Fat: 0 g, Cholesterol: 0 mg, Calcium:
169 mg, Sodium: 728 mg.

NOTE: The sodium in this dish is a little high, but it's worth it here for all the fiber
and other nutrients. If you can be satisfied with half the amount of salt, then the
sodium drops to 610 mg.

Tomato-Basil Mini Pizzas

These kid-tested pizzas will be a hit with the entire family.

MAKES 4 PIZZAS (SERVES 2 ADULTS, OR 4 YOUNG CHILDREN)

- 4 tomatoes, peeled, seeded, and diced
- 1 tablespoon chopped basil
- 1 clove minced garlic
- Dash of salt
- 4 Mini Harvest Wheat Flatout Flatbreads (70 calories each)
- 6 ounces part-skim mozzarella, grated

Preheat oven to 400 degrees F.

In a saucepan combine tomatoes, basil, garlic, and salt. Cook over medium heat, stirring frequently, until most of the liquid is gone, approximately 10 minutes.

Spray a cookie sheet with oil spray. Lay flatbreads on cookie sheet and spread 2 tablespoons of sauce on each. Sprinkle a quarter of the cheese on top of each pizza.

Cook until cheese is bubbly and flatbreads are crispy, approximately 10 minutes. Serve immediately.

PER PIZZA, ABOUT: Calories: 201, Protein: 15 g, Carbohydrate: 19 g, Dietary Fiber: 5 g, Total Fat: 8 g, Saturated Fat: 4 g, Cholesterol: 27 mg, Calcium: 347 mg, Sodium: 498 mg.

Vegetable and Grain Side Dishes

Broccoli Rabe with Pine Nuts and Currants

Broccoli rabe is a slightly stronger-tasting member of the broccoli family. If you can't find it, substitute regular broccoli or broccolini, a hybrid of Chinese kale and broccoli.

SERVES 4

- 1 bunch of broccoli rabe (about 1 pound)
- 1 tablespoon olive oil

   2 cloves garlic, chopped

   3 tablespoons pine nuts

   ¾ cup water

   ¼ cup currants

   Salt and freshly ground pepper

Rinse the broccoli rabe. Trim away the dry ends of the stalks and discard. Cut the stalks into 1-inch pieces.

Heat the olive oil in a large skillet over a medium flame. Sauté the garlic and pine nuts until they begin to color, about 1 minute. Add the water and broccoli rabe, tossing gently. Add the currants and stir to combine.

Simmer, covered, until the stalks are tender throughout, about 10 minutes. Season with salt and freshly ground pepper.

PER SERVING, ABOUT: Calories: 129, Protein: 4 g, Carbohydrate: 11 g, Dietary Fiber: 3 g, Total Fat: 8 g, Saturated Fat: 1 g, Cholesterol: 0 mg, Calcium: 127 mg, Sodium: 30 mg.

Wilted Greens with Garlic and Sesame Oil

This recipe calls for spinach, but chard, kale, or any other green will also work fine.

SERVES 4

   Nonstick cooking spray

   1 teaspoon sesame oil

   4 cloves garlic, minced

   20 ounces spinach leaves, washed well

   1 teaspoon rice vinegar, or to taste

   Salt and freshly ground pepper

Spray a large skillet with cooking spray and place it over a medium-high flame. Add the sesame oil and garlic, and sauté until the garlic begins to soften, about 30 seconds. Add the spinach and vinegar, and sauté until the spinach is just wilted, about 2 minutes. Season with salt and pepper.

PER SERVING, ABOUT: Calories: 54, Protein: 4 g, Carbohydrate: 7 g, Dietary
Fiber: 3 g, Total Fat: 2 g, Saturated Fat: 0 g, Cholesterol: 0 mg, Calcium: 146 mg,
Sodium: 132 mg.

Green Beans with Tomatoes and Feta

This is a fresh take on the classic green bean casserole.

SERVES 8

> Two 7.4-ounce boxes Cascadian Farm frozen organic French-cut green
>   beans with toasted almonds
> 1 tablespoon olive oil
> 1 medium onion, sliced
> 2 cloves garlic, finely chopped
> One 14½-ounce can diced tomatoes, such as Muir Glen organic, undrained
> 1 teaspoon chopped fresh oregano leaves or ½ teaspoon of dried oregano
>   leaves
> ⅛ teaspoon crushed red pepper, if desired
> ⅓ cup crumbled feta cheese

Cook beans as directed on box, reserving almonds; drain.

Meanwhile, in a 10-inch skillet, heat the olive oil over medium heat. Cook
the onion and garlic in the olive oil for 3 to 4 minutes, stirring frequently,
until the onion is crisp-tender. Stir in the tomatoes, oregano, and red
pepper. Heat until boiling. Reduce the heat; simmer, uncovered, for about
5 minutes, stirring occasionally, until thickened and most of the liquid is
evaporated.

Spoon the drained beans onto a serving platter; top with the tomato
mixture. Sprinkle with feta cheese and the reserved almonds.

PER SERVING, ABOUT: Calories: 80, Protein: 2 g, Carbohydrate: 8 g, Dietary
Fiber: 1 g, Total Fat: 5 g, Saturated Fat: 1 g, Cholesterol: 5 mg, Calcium: 65 mg,
Sodium: 279 mg.

Roasted Fennel with Parmesan

This dish is a nice accompaniment to the Chicken with Artichokes and
Melted Lemons on page 234.

SERVES 4

> Nonstick cooking spray
>
> 2 fennel bulbs (about 1¾–2 pounds), cut horizontally into ½-inch-thick
> slices
>
> 3 tablespoons toasted whole grain bread crumbs*
>
> ¼ cup grated Parmesan cheese
>
> Salt and freshly ground pepper to taste
>
> 2 tablespoons extra-virgin olive oil

Preheat the oven to 375 degrees F. Lightly spray a 9 x 9-inch baking dish
with nonstick cooking spray. Place the sliced fennel in a dish and sprinkle
with bread crumbs, Parmesan, salt, and pepper. Drizzle with the olive oil.
Roast until the fennel is tender and the top layer is starting to brown, about
1 hour. Season with more salt and pepper, if necessary.

*For the bread crumbs, remove crust from 1 slice of whole grain bread. Tear the
slice into bite-size pieces (about ⅓–½ cup in torn pieces) and toast them lightly in a
400-degree-F. heated oven for 10 to 12 minutes, stirring once or twice to toast evenly.
Remove and let cool. When cool, process in a food processor or blender until fine.

PER SERVING, ABOUT: Calories: 143, Protein: 6 g, Carbohydrate: 12 g, Dietary
Fiber: 4 g, Total Fat: 9 g, Saturated Fat: 2 g, Cholesterol: 6 mg, Calcium: 137 mg,
Sodium: 195 mg.

Sautéed Sugar Snap Peas with Ginger

Fresh sugar snap peas are one of spring's delights. In other seasons, frozen
peas work well in this dish, too.

SERVES 4

> 3 teaspoons sesame oil
>
> 1 tablespoon ginger, minced
>
> 2 teaspoons garlic, minced

2 pints (about 5 cups) fresh or frozen sugar snap peas, washed, ends trimmed

3 tablespoons fat-free chicken broth, such as Health Valley fat-free chicken broth or Pacific Foods low-sodium chicken broth

In a medium skillet over a medium-low flame, heat the sesame oil and sauté the ginger and garlic for 1 minute, stirring. Raise the flame to medium, add the peas and chicken broth, and continue to cook until the peas are tender but not too soft, about 2 minutes. Serve warm.

PER SERVING, ABOUT: Calories: 117, Protein: 7 g, Carbohydrate: 15 g, Dietary Fiber: 6 g, Total Fat: 4 g, Saturated Fat: 1 g, Cholesterol: 0 mg, Calcium: 87 mg, Sodium: 9 mg.

Herbed Barley with Roasted Cherry Tomatoes and Feta

You may want to double this recipe—the leftovers make a great lunch.

SERVES 6

1½ cups cherry or grape tomato halves

2 teaspoons olive oil

Salt and freshly ground pepper

2 cups water

¾ teaspoon salt

1 cup pearl barley, sorted and rinsed

1 tablespoon fresh sage, finely chopped

1 tablespoon fresh oregano, finely chopped

1 tablespoon fresh Italian parsley, chopped

¼ cup crumbled feta cheese

Lemon Vinaigrette

Juice and zest of 1 lemon

1 small clove garlic, finely minced

2 tablespoons olive oil

Preheat oven to 425 degrees F. In a baking dish, toss the tomatoes with the olive oil, season with salt and pepper, and roast, shaking often, until the tomatoes are lightly browned on the outside, 10 to 15 minutes.

Bring the water and ¾ teaspoon salt to a boil in a medium saucepan over medium heat. Slowly add the barley. Cover, reduce the heat to low, and cook for 30 to 40 minutes, or until the barley is tender and the water is absorbed. Transfer to a bowl and cool.

Meanwhile, combine the lemon vinaigrette ingredients in a small bowl and whisk to blend. Add to the barley and toss to combine.

Add the roasted tomatoes, chopped herbs, and crumbled cheese, and toss again.

PER SERVING, ABOUT: Calories: 200, Protein: 5 g, Carbohydrate: 29 g, Dietary Fiber: 6 g, Total Fat: 8 g, Saturated Fat: 2 g, Cholesterol: 5 mg, Calcium: 60 mg, Sodium: 369 mg.

Grilled Eggplant Stacks with Bulgur, Tomatoes, and Feta

The finished result of this beautiful dish makes it look complicated. In reality, it's a snap to make.

SERVES 4

- 2 cups fat-free reduced-sodium chicken or vegetable broth, such as Health Valley fat-free chicken broth, Pacific Foods low-sodium chicken broth, or Health Valley fat-free vegetable broth
- 1 cup bulgur wheat
- 2 medium eggplants
- Olive oil cooking spray
- Eight ½-inch-thick tomato slices
- 4 ounces feta cheese
- 3 tablespoons chopped kalamata olives
- 2 tablespoons chopped fresh basil or mint
- ½ teaspoon grated lemon zest
- Salt and freshly ground pepper
- Basil or mint sprigs, for garnish

Bring the broth to a boil in a medium saucepan. Slowly stir in the bulgur. Reduce the heat to low, cover the pan, and cook until broth is absorbed, about 15 minutes. Keep warm.

Slice the eggplants crosswise into ½-inch slices. You will need 12 slices of similar diameter. Arrange the slices in a single layer on a baking sheet and coat the eggplant lightly with some of the cooking spray. Turn the slices over and spray again.

Cook the eggplant over medium-hot coals or on a preheated grill pan until tender, about 5 minutes on each side. Set aside and keep warm.

Place a cooking spray–coated sheet of foil big enough to hold the tomato slices on the grill. Arrange the tomatoes on the foil. Cover the grill and cook until the tomatoes are heated through, about 5 minutes. Alternatively, the tomatoes can be heated on a baking sheet in a 350-degree-F. oven.

Meanwhile, stir the feta, olives, basil or mint, and lemon zest into the hot bulgur. Season with salt and pepper.

To assemble, place 1 eggplant slice on each of four warm plates. Top with 1 tomato slice and some of the bulgur mixture. Repeat. Top each stack with 1 more eggplant slice. Garnish each stack with a basil or mint sprig.

PER SERVING, ABOUT: Calories: 235, Protein: 9 g, Carbohydrate: 28 g, Dietary Fiber: 12 g, Total Fat: 11 g, Saturated Fat: 5 g, Cholesterol: 25 mg, Calcium: 177 mg, Sodium: 445 mg.

Quinoa with Corn, Peppers, and Cilantro

Quinoa has double the protein of rice and a pleasant bit of crunch.

SERVES 4

> ½ cup uncooked quinoa
>
> 1 cup water
>
> 1 cup diced red bell pepper
>
> 1 cup frozen corn kernels, such as Cascadian Farm organic Super Sweet, cooked
>
> ½ cup chopped red onion
>
> ½ cup chopped cilantro
>
> Juice and grated zest of 1 lime
>
> ¼ teaspoon ground cumin
>
> 3 tablespoons extra-virgin olive oil
>
> Salt and freshly ground pepper

Place the quinoa in a fine strainer and rinse thoroughly with cold water. In a small saucepan, bring 1 cup of water and the quinoa to a boil. Reduce the flame to low, cover, and cook for 15 minutes, or until the grains are translucent and the germ has spiraled out from each grain. Transfer to a large bowl and chill. Add the bell pepper, corn, onion, and cilantro to the chilled quinoa. Toss to combine.

In a small bowl, whisk together the lime juice, lime zest, cumin, and olive oil. Pour over the quinoa mixture and toss well. Season with salt and pepper.

PER SERVING, ABOUT: Calories: 228, Protein: 5 g, Carbohydrate: 29 g, Dietary Fiber: 4 g, Total Fat: 12 g, Saturated Fat: 2 g, Cholesterol: 0 mg, Calcium: 30 mg, Sodium: 11 mg.

Farro with Spinach and Cherry Tomatoes

Farro is a grain popular in Italy that has a firm, chewy texture. If you can't find it locally, try www.igourmet.com.

  1 cup farro or barley
  1 tablespoon olive oil
  1 small onion, chopped
  2 cloves garlic, minced
  1 cup cherry tomatoes
  6 ounces baby spinach, washed well
  Salt and freshly ground pepper
  4 teaspoons grated Parmesan cheese

Cook the farro in 2 quarts of boiling water until tender, 10 to 12 minutes.

Meanwhile, heat the olive oil in a large skillet or pot set over a medium-high flame. Add the onion and cook, stirring often, until the onion begins to soften, about 5 minutes. Add the garlic and cherry tomatoes and sauté just until the tomato skins start to burst, about 3 minutes.

When the farro is cooked, drain and stir it into the tomato mixture along with the spinach. Stir to combine. Remove from heat, cover, and let stand for 1 minute, or until spinach is wilted. Season with salt and pepper. Serve sprinkled with Parmesan cheese.

PER SERVING, ABOUT: Calories: 227, Protein: 8 g, Carbohydrate: 39 g, Dietary Fiber: 10 g, Total Fat: 5 g, Saturated Fat: 1 g, Cholesterol: 2 mg, Calcium: 84 mg, Sodium: 69 mg.

Rosemary Roasted Sweet Potatoes

Once you taste these, you'll never eat sweet potatoes with marshmallows again!

SERVES 4

> 2 pounds sweet potatoes, peeled (about 2 large)
>
> ¼ cup walnuts, finely chopped
>
> 2 tablespoons extra-virgin olive oil
>
> 1 tablespoon chopped fresh rosemary
>
> 1 teaspoon minced garlic
>
> ½ teaspoon kosher salt
>
> ⅛ teaspoon black pepper
>
> Nonstick cooking spray

Place the potatoes in a large saucepan, cover with cold water, and bring to a boil. Reduce the heat and cook, covered, at a low boil until the potatoes start to soften, about 15 minutes.

While the potatoes are cooking, mix together the walnuts, olive oil, rosemary, garlic, salt, and pepper in a bowl. Set aside.

When the potatoes are done, remove and let cool, 10 to 15 minutes. Preheat the oven to 425 degrees F. Slice the potatoes into ½-inch-thick rounds and place in a single layer on a large baking sheet coated with nonstick cooking spray. Spread the walnut mixture evenly over each sweet potato round, and bake until the topping turns golden and the potatoes are soft, about 25 minutes.

PER SERVING, ABOUT: Calories: 305, Protein: 5 g, Carbohydrate: 47 g, Dietary Fiber: 7 g, Total Fat: 12 g, Saturated Fat: 1 g, Cholesterol: 0 mg, Calcium: 78 mg, Sodium: 365 mg.

DESSERTS

Banana-Walnut Polenta Pudding

SERVES 6

¾ cup polenta or cornmeal

¾ teaspoon cinnamon

5 cups water

1 tablespoon safflower oil

½ cup chopped walnuts

2 ripe bananas, peeled and sliced

½ cup maple syrup or honey

In a large bowl, mix the polenta and cinnamon.

In a saucepan, bring water to a boil. Slowly stir in the polenta mixture. Return to a boil. Reduce the heat, then cover and simmer for 30 to 40 minutes, until the polenta is very soft, stirring frequently. If the mixture becomes too thick, stir in additional water.

Meanwhile, in a skillet, heat the safflower oil over a medium flame. Add the walnuts and toast them, stirring, for 2 minutes.

Add the banana slices and cook for 2 minutes longer, until the bananas begin to brown and soften. Stir in the syrup and cook for 1 minute longer.

When the polenta is cooked, remove from the heat and stir in the walnuts and bananas. Serve warm.

PER SERVING, ABOUT: Calories: 253, Protein: 3 g, Carbohydrate: 42 g, Dietary Fiber: 3 g, Total Fat: 9 g, Saturated Fat: 1 g, Cholesterol: 0 mg, Calcium: 34 mg, Sodium: 4 mg.

Naked Peach Pies

If you like peach pie, you'll like this lower-calorie (but still sweet and yummy) version.

SERVES 6

1½ cups Cascadian Farm Organic Purely O's or Cheerios

3 tablespoons brown sugar (for extra flavor, try muscovado brown sugar)

3 tablespoons chopped pecans

2 tablespoons oat bran

3 tablespoons soy nut butter

One 10-ounce package frozen sliced peaches, such as Cascadian Farm organic, thawed

1 teaspoon freshly squeezed lemon juice

½ teaspoon ground cinnamon

½ teaspoon ground nutmeg

Preheat the oven to 350 degrees F.

Place the Purely O's in a 1-gallon zippered plastic bag. Using a rolling pin or can of soup, crush the O's. Place in a small bowl, add the brown sugar, and blend with the pecans, oat bran, and soy nut butter. Work the mixture with your fingers until crumbly.

In a 9-inch pie plate, toss the peaches with the lemon juice, cinnamon, and nutmeg. Sprinkle with the topping. Bake until the fruit is bubbly and topping is browned, about 25 minutes.

PER SERVING, ABOUT: Calories: 140, Protein: 4 g, Carbohydrate: 21 g, Dietary Fiber: 3 g, Total Fat: 6 g, Saturated Fat: 1 g, Cholesterol: 0 mg, Calcium: 66 mg, Sodium: 107 mg.

Blueberry Yogurt Coffee Cake

This coffee cake is a nice addition to brunch or can be served as dessert.

SERVES 12

　　Nonstick cooking spray

　　1½ cups unbleached all-purpose flour

　　½ cup whole wheat flour

　　¾ teaspoon baking powder

　　¾ teaspoon baking soda

　　¼ teaspoon salt

　　1 teaspoon cinnamon

　　1¼ cups nonfat plain yogurt, such as Colombo

　　⅓ cup canola oil

　　⅓ cup brown sugar (for extra flavor, try muscovado brown sugar)

　　1 whole egg

　　2 egg whites

　　1½ teaspoons vanilla extract

　　1½ cups blueberries, fresh or frozen and thawed

　　¾ cup Low-Fat Winter Fruit Granola (see recipe on page 197) or store-
　　　　bought low-fat granola

Preheat the oven to 350 degrees F. Coat a 10-inch round cake pan with
nonstick cooking spray.

In a large bowl, combine the flours, baking powder, baking soda, salt, and
cinnamon. Whisk to combine.

In a medium bowl, combine the yogurt, canola oil, brown sugar, egg, egg
whites, and vanilla. Whisk to blend thoroughly.

Make a well in the dry ingredients. Pour in the yogurt mixture, and stir just
until the dry ingredients are moistened. Gently fold in the blueberries.

Transfer to the prepared pan. Sprinkle the granola evenly over the top.

Bake until the center of the cake springs back when lightly tapped with your
finger, about 30 minutes. Serve warm.

PER SERVING, ABOUT: Calories: 203, Protein: 6 g, Carbohydrate: 29 g, Dietary
Fiber: 2 g, Total Fat: 7 g, Saturated Fat: 1 g, Cholesterol: 18 mg, Calcium: 84 mg,
Sodium: 133 mg.

Roasted Peaches with Ricotta and Almonds

These peaches are beautiful to look at and absolutely simple to make.

SERVES 6

> 3 large ripe peaches
>
> Nonstick cooking spray
>
> 1 cup part-skim ricotta cheese
>
> 3 tablespoons honey
>
> 1 teaspoon freshly squeezed lemon juice
>
> 1 teaspoon vanilla extract
>
> ½ teaspoon almond extract
>
> ¼ teaspoon cinnamon
>
> Pinch salt
>
> ¼ cup toasted sliced almonds

Preheat the oven to 400 degrees F.

Drop the peaches into a pot of boiling water, turn off the heat, and let stand for 1 minute. Drain. When peaches are cool enough to handle, slip the skins off. Cut the peaches in half and remove pits.

With a sharp knife, cut a thin slice from the rounded side of each peach half and arrange the peach halves, pit-side up, in a pie plate coated with nonstick cooking spray. Mince the thin slices and mash them slightly with the side of the knife.

In a bowl, combine the ricotta cheese, mashed peaches, honey, lemon juice, vanilla and almond extracts, cinnamon, and salt. Stir to blend. Gently fold in the almonds.

Mound some of the ricotta mixture into cavity of each peach. Bake for 10 minutes. Serve warm.

PER SERVING, ABOUT: Calories: 161, Protein: 7 g, Carbohydrate: 20 g, Dietary Fiber: 2 g, Total Fat: 7 g, Saturated Fat: 2 g, Cholesterol: 13 mg, Calcium: 135 mg, Sodium: 52 mg.

Apple Rhubarb Walnut Crisp

Tart rhubarb gives this classic recipe a slight tang.

SERVES 6–8

Filling

3 large Red or Golden Delicious apples, peeled, cored, and cut into ½-inch pieces, about 4 cups

1 pound rhubarb, cut into ½-inch pieces (about 3 cups)

2 tablespoons packed brown sugar

2 tablespoons whole wheat flour

1 teaspoon vanilla extract

½ teaspoon ground cinnamon

Crisp Topping

½ cup walnuts, very finely chopped

¼ cup packed brown sugar

¼ cup quick-cooking oats

¼ cup whole wheat flour

½ teaspoon ground cinnamon

⅛ teaspoon salt

2 tablespoons canola oil

Preheat the oven to 400 degrees F. Combine the apples, rhubarb, brown sugar, flour, vanilla extract, and cinnamon in a large bowl and toss to coat. Place the apple mixture in an 8 x 8-inch baking dish and set aside.

To make the topping, combine the walnuts, brown sugar, oats, flour, cinnamon, and salt in a medium bowl. Add the canola oil and stir until the dry ingredients are well coated.

Spread the topping evenly over the fruit mixture. Bake for 40 to 45 minutes, or until the fruit is tender and the topping is golden brown (cover with foil if the topping browns too quickly).

PER SERVING, ABOUT (⅙ OF THE RECIPE PRESENTED FIRST, FOLLOWED BY NUMBERS FOR ⅛ OF THE RECIPE): Calories: 287 (215), Protein: 4 g (3 g), Carbohydrate: 46 g (34 g), Dietary Fiber: 5 g (4 g), Total Fat: 12 g (9 g), Saturated Fat: 1 g (1 g), Cholesterol: 0 mg, Calcium: 103 mg (77 mg), Sodium: 58 mg (43 mg).

Triple-Berry Granola Crisp

I use Cascadian Farm organic frozen fruit to make this easy crisp because it's so flavorful. It's as close as you can get to eating fresh-picked berries.

SERVES 9

>   One 10-ounce bag frozen blueberries
>
>   One 10-ounce bag frozen strawberries
>
>   One 10-ounce bag frozen raspberries
>
>   ¼ cup sugar
>
>   2 tablespoons all-purpose flour
>
>   1½ cups Cascadian Farm organic oat and honey granola, or other granola

Preheat the oven to 375 degrees F. In an ungreased 8-inch-square (2-quart) glass baking dish, stir together the frozen berries, sugar, and flour until the fruit is coated.

Bake for 20 minutes. Stir; sprinkle with granola.

Bake for 15 to 20 minutes longer or until light golden brown and bubbly. Let stand for 5 to 10 minutes before serving.

PER SERVING, ABOUT: Calories: 127, Protein: 2 g, Carbohydrate: 28 g, Dietary Fiber: 4 g, Total Fat: 2 g, Saturated Fat: 0 g, Cholesterol: 0 mg, Calcium: 24 mg, Sodium: 31 mg.

Hazelnut Biscotti

16 BISCOTTI, 1 PER SERVING

Nonstick cooking spray

3 tablespoons light olive oil, such as Bertolli Extra-Light Tasting Olive Oil

1 egg, lightly beaten

⅓ cup hazelnuts, toasted, skinned, and coarsely chopped

¾ cup all-purpose flour

¼ cup firmly packed light brown sugar

2 tablespoons granulated sugar

½ teaspoon ground cinnamon

½ teaspoon baking powder

¼ teaspoon salt

Preheat the oven to 350 degrees F. Spray a cookie sheet with nonstick cooking spray; set aside.

In a small bowl, combine the olive oil and egg until well blended.

In a large bowl, combine the hazelnuts, flour, sugars, cinnamon, baking powder, and salt. Stir in the egg-oil mixture to form a dough, kneading by hand as needed. Form into 9 x 3 x ½-inch log. Place on prepared pan.

Bake for 20 minutes. Remove from oven and place on wire rack; cool slightly, about 20 minutes. Return to oven and bake an additional 10 minutes. Slice diagonally into ½-inch-thick slices. Reduce oven temperature to 330 degrees F. Bake, cut side down, an additional 15 minutes. Cool completely on wire rack.

PER SERVING, ABOUT: Calories: 83, Protein: 1 g, Carbohydrate: 10 g, Dietary Fiber: 0 g, Total Fat: 4 g, Saturated Fat: 1 g, Cholesterol: 13 mg, Calcium: 18 mg, Sodium: 58 mg.

Peachy Pops

A wonderful, creamy smoothie on a stick.

SERVES 10

> 1½ cups 8th Continent vanilla soymilk
>
> 2 cups frozen sliced peaches, partially thawed
>
> 3 tablespoons honey
>
> Ten 3-ounce paper cups
>
> Foil
>
> 10 craft sticks (flat wooden sticks with round ends)

Place the soymilk, peaches, and honey in a blender. Cover; blend on high for about 1 minute, or until smooth.

Place the paper cups in a rectangular pan; pour the mixture into paper cups. Cover the top of each cup with foil; insert a stick through the foil into each pop. Freeze for 2 to 3 hours, or until firm.

PER SERVING, ABOUT: Calories: 56, Protein: 1 g, Carbohydrate: 12 g, Dietary Fiber: 1 g, Total Fat: 0 g, Saturated Fat: 0 g, Cholesterol: 0 mg, Calcium: 48 mg, Sodium: 26 mg.

CALCIUM-RICH SNACKS

Mocha Cooler

A healthy take on the frozen blended drinks available at coffee cafés.

SERVES 2

> 1 medium banana, cut into chunks
>
> 2 cups 8th Continent Light chocolate soymilk
>
> 2 teaspoons instant coffee granules or crystals
>
> ½ teaspoon vanilla extract
>
> 1 cup ice cubes

In a blender, place all the ingredients except ice cubes. Cover; blend on high speed for about 15 seconds, or until smooth.

Add ice cubes. Cover; blend for about 15 seconds longer, or until blended.

Pour into 2 glasses. Serve immediately.

PER SERVING, ABOUT: Calories: 148, Protein: 8 g, Carbohydrate: 26 g, Dietary Fiber: 2 g, Total Fat: 2 g, Saturated Fat: 0 g, Cholesterol: 0 mg, Calcium: 304 mg, Sodium: 181 mg.

Vanilla Caramel Truffle Latte

A rich, creamy treat for tea lovers.

SERVES 2

> 2 cups 1 percent milk
>
> 1 cup water
>
> 2 cinnamon sticks
>
> 3 Lipton Premium Pyramid Vanilla Caramel Truffle tea bags
>
> 3 teaspoons of sugar

In a 1-quart saucepan, bring the milk, water, and cinnamon sticks just to a boil. Remove the saucepan from heat and add the tea bags. Brew for 3 minutes; remove the tea bags and cinnamon. Stir in the sugar and serve immediately.

PER SERVING, ABOUT: Calories: 128, Protein: 8 g, Carbohydrate: 19 g, Dietary Fiber: 0 g, Total Fat: 2 g, Saturated Fat: 2 g, Cholesterol: 12 mg, Calcium: 290 mg, Sodium: 111 mg.

Iced Vanilla Soy Latte

It's hard to believe that these luscious drinks have only 118 calories per serving.

SERVES 2

> ½ cup ground espresso or French roast coffee
>
> 1½ cups water
>
> 2 cups 8th Continent vanilla soymilk
>
> 2 teaspoons caramel or chocolate fat-free topping
>
> Ice cubes, to taste
>
> Sugar, if desired

Using a drip coffeemaker, brew coffee with water as directed by coffee-maker manufacturer. Stir the soymilk into the coffee. Drizzle the insides of two large glasses with topping. Fill glasses with ice cubes as desired. Pour coffee mixture over ice. Sweeten to taste with sugar.

PER SERVING, ABOUT: Calories: 118, Protein: 6 g, Carbohydrate: 16 g, Dietary Fiber: 0 g, Total Fat: 3 g, Saturated Fat: 0 g, Cholesterol: 0 mg, Calcium: 305 mg, Sodium: 195 mg.

Berry Smoothies

Raspberries also work nicely in this smoothie.

SERVES 2

> 1¼ cups 8th Continent vanilla soymilk
>
> 1 cup frozen unsweetened blueberries, such as Cascadian Farm organic
>
> One 6-ounce container Yoplait Original French Vanilla yogurt

Place ingredients in a blender and blend until smooth.

PER SERVING, ABOUT: Calories: 187, Protein: 7 g, Carbohydrate: 33 g, Dietary Fiber: 2 g, Total Fat: 3 g, Saturated Fat: 1 g, Cholesterol: 5 mg, Calcium: 294 mg, Sodium: 147 mg.

METRIC EQUIVALENCIES

LIQUID EQUIVALENCIES

CUSTOMARY	METRIC
1/4 teaspoon	1.25 milliliters
1/2 teaspoon	2.5 milliliters
1 teaspoon	5 milliliters
1 tablespoon	15 milliliters
1 fluid ounce	30 milliliters
1/4 cup	60 milliliters
1/3 cup	80 milliliters
1/2 cup	120 milliliters
1 cup	240 milliliters
1 pint (2 cups)	480 milliliters
1 quart (4 cups)	960 milliliters (.96 liter)
1 gallon (4 quarts)	3.84 liters

DRY MEASURE EQUIVALENCIES

CUSTOMARY	METRIC
1 ounce (by weight)	28 grams
1/4 pound (4 ounces)	114 grams
1 pound (16 ounces)	454 grams
2.2 pounds	1 kilogram (1,000 grams)

OVEN TEMPERATURE EQUIVALENCIES

DESCRIPTION	°FAHRENHEIT	°CELSIUS
Cool	200	90
Very slow	250	120
Slow	300–325	150–160
Moderately slow	325–350	160–180
Moderate	350–375	180–190
Moderately hot	375–400	190–200
Hot	400–450	200–230
Very hot	450–500	230–260

GENERAL INDEX

RECIPE INDEX

ABOUT THE AUTHOR

▶ Bob Greene is an exercise physiologist and certified personal trainer specializing in fitness, metabolism, and weight loss. He holds a master's degree from the University of Arizona and is a member of the American College of Sports Medicine and the American Council on Exercise. For the past seventeen years, he has worked with clients and consulted on the design and management of fitness, spa, and sports medicine programs. Bob has been a frequent guest on the *Oprah Winfrey Show.* He is also a contributing writer and editor for *O, the Oprah magazine* and writes articles on health and fitness for Oprah.com. Greene is an ambassador for McDonald's Balanced Active Lifestyles Initiative and the bestselling author of *Bob Greene's Total Body Makeover, Bob Greene's Total Body Makeover Daily Journal, Get with the Program!, The Get with the Program! Daily Journal, The Get with the Program! Guide to Good Eating,* and *The Get with the Program! Guide to Fast Food & Family Restaurants.*

You can visit Bob Green at his website, www.thebestlife.com.

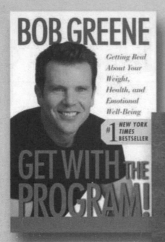
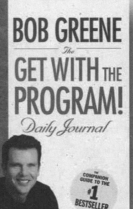
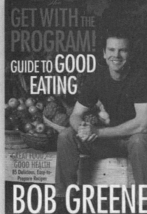
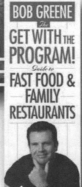

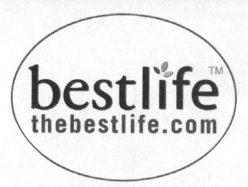